THIRD OPINION

OPINION

SECOND EDITION

An International Directory to Alternative Therapy Centers for the Treatment and Prevention of Cancer and Other Degenerative Diseases

JOHN M. FINK

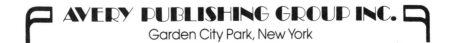

AVERY PUBLISHING GROUP INC.
Garden City Park, New York

The publisher does not advocate the use of any particular form of health care but believes the information presented in this book should be available to the public. Treatments always involve some risk; therefore, the author and publisher disclaim responsibility for any ill effects or harmful consequences resulting from the use of any treatments listed in this book. The reader should feel free to consult a physician or other qualified health professional. It is a sign of wisdom, not cowardice, to seek an expert opinion.

Cover Design: Rudy Shur and Martin Hochberg
In-House Editor: Arthur Vidro
Typesetting: Multifacit Graphics Inc.; Keyport, New Jersey

Library of Congress Cataloging-in-Publication Data

Fink, John M.
    Third opinion : an international directory to alternative therapy
centers for the treatment and prevention of cancer and other
degenerative diseases / John M. Fink. — 2nd ed.
      p. cm.
    Includes bibliographical references and index.
    ISBN 0-89529-503-2 (pbk.)
    1. Cancer—Alternative treatment—Directories.   2. Alternative
medicine—Directories.   I. Title.
    [DNLM: 1. Alternative Medicine—directories.   2. Cancer Care
Facilities—directories.   3. Hospitals, Special—directories.
  4. Neoplasms—prevention & control—directories.   5. Neoplasms—
therapy—directories.   6. Physicians—directories.   QZ 22.1 F499t]
RC271.A62F56   1992
362.1'96994—dc20
DNLM/DLC
for Library of Congress   91-41082
                                          CIP

Printed in the United States of America

10 9 8 7 6 5 4 3 2

Contents

To Phoebe and Sharkey

Preface

My wife Sharkey and I had been married almost ten years before we felt we were ready to take on the responsibility of having a child. Phoebe, our little girl, brought us great light and happiness from the moment she was born. She was the best thing that ever happened to us, and when she was two and a half and doctors first diagnosed her as having a rare form of cancer, there wasn't anything we wouldn't have done to save her.

When the cancer recurred four months after a very difficult operation, and the conventional treatments of chemotherapy and radiation offered no hope (based on all previously recorded similar cases), we were willing to pursue anything that would offer a glimpse of hope as long as it wouldn't needlessly interfere with the quality of her life.

As Sharkey was seven months pregnant, we called our old Lamaze teacher to enroll in her class. Of course, we told her about Phoebe. She told me to call an actor that I'd been in a television series with and whom she had known through her classes. She said that he had been in similar circumstances with his mother about a year earlier and had turned to a complementary therapy.

I called him the next day, and he put us in touch with the Cancer Control Society, an organization in Los Angeles that provides information about unconventional therapies. They were very helpful in laying out some options among the alternative programs, telling us many of the things we needed to know to make a decision and showing us how we could go about reaching various clinics, many of which were outside this country.

After numerous telephone calls, we chose a nutritional therapy for our daughter. Because we wanted the guidance of a doctor to help us get started, we went to a clinic in Mexico that specialized in this therapy under the auspices of Mexican doctors. There we were encouraged to undergo the therapy as a family to improve our health and prevent any health problems in our son, Andy, who had just been born.

Almost immediately after starting the program, Sharkey and I reaped health benefits. Sharkey's hay fever and chronic sinusitis cleared up completely, and she remains symptom free. My chronic hay fever and mild asthma, which had plagued me for 23 years and for which I, like Sharkey, had been receiving conventional treatment, went away. We began to believe in the relationship between diet and well-being. (In those days, the late 1970s, it wasn't even acknowledged by United States medical doctors that there was a link between most diseases and what you ate.) Our faith was reinforced at the clinic when we observed some patients with advanced cases of cancer, rheumatoid arthritis, diabetes, and heart disease responding well to the same diet.

Continuing with this comprehensive but demanding therapy over the next year and a half proved at times very stressful for us and our little daughter. After a few months, there were indications that the therapy on its own wasn't stopping the cancer. We tried introducing a few other harmless but potentially beneficial foods, herbs, and vitamins into Phoebe's diet. During this time we were greatly helped by all the information that came to us and by the assistance and support of others, who seemed to appear miraculously in times of need. Among them were people who showed us paths of healing in herbs, naturopathy, homeopathy, Eastern medicine, imagery, and meditation, just to mention a few. These people greatly enriched our lives.

In having taken the responsibility for Phoebe's well-being, we found ourselves learning to take responsibility for our own lives and, in doing so, tapping strengths and inner resources that serve us today. And during Phoebe's last months, we were very grateful to be able to help her to be free from the pain, suffering, and loneliness that often accompany cancer.

During the time Phoebe was still alive, we collected an enormous amount of information on complementary programs and talked with many recovered cancer patients. Piecing it all together wasn't easy. As our days were occupied in working on the therapy, we stayed awake late at night reading everything we could get our hands on concerning alternatives. Sharkey blazed the trails. She would read well after I had dropped off to sleep in exhaustion.

At some point in that year and a half, I had a vision of this directory. I knew that a guidebook would have been a tremendous help to us, and I knew that I would write it one day. Although I hadn't counted on its taking eight years from conceptualization to completion, I am convinced that there is a greater need than ever for this book.

I must pay tribute to Sue Carlan, who came as a college student to help me when I first rolled up my sleeves on this project. She spent hours and hours working on the various listings and showed courage where it failed me in fearlessly attacking my new computer and leading me gently along into this new technology. Her impish humor and high spirits equaled her dedication to and faith in this book, and I shall always be grateful to her.

After Sue left, James Rojas, already a wiz on the Macintosh, came to help. He showed me new ways of organizing the material and replaced Sue in working diligently on the listings in front of the electronic box. I am very appreciative.

My confidence in this project was greatly increased as a result of the time and commitment that Rudy Shur, managing editor of Avery Publishing Group, put into it. With Steven Blauer's input and good judgment, Rudy guided me toward better organizing and presenting this material. Additionally, editors Joanne Abrams and Laura Iacono of Avery kept throwing me the lifesaver. And Arthur Vidro was invaluable on the revised edition. I was lucky to find them all.

Deep appreciation goes to Sharkey for all her help and constructive comments. I couldn't have done this without her.

And no amount of thanks will do in crediting Michael Lerner for the time, encouragement, and support he showed for this undertaking since we first traveled together, looking at the clinics in 1982. His continual support of my work has meant a great deal to me.

For encouraging me to get a computer and do this book years ago, I am indebted to Stephan Schwartz, who was always there when I needed him and who spoon-fed me on the computer when I needed it. He also gave me many fine suggestions.

For reading the original manuscript and giving me many specific ways to improve this work, I thank John August, Grace Aldworth, Lorraine Rosenthal, Hal Card, Shirley Tyler, Jerry Freedman, and Dr. Walter Taylor.

For helping and heartening me, thanks to my other traveling companion, Dr. Sandra McLanahan, and to Ann Cinquina, Peter Barry Chowka, Marie Steinmeyer, Tom Atherton, Frank Wiewel, and the late Betty Lee Morales.

For giving me guidance in getting a publisher, I owe a debt to Tom Monte, Ann Fransen, Hope Innes, and Ken Cohen.

To G. Haro, for having given me the Macintosh that made all this possible, "Muchícimas gracias, Señor."

To the Reverend Jeffrey Duncan, Rabbi Wydoff, and Swami Satchidananda, for their inspiration, I am truly beholden.

Finally, to those who really deserve the ultimate accolades: thank you, Mother, for having put up with me all those years; thank you Sharkey, Andy, and Lily for putting up with me all these years; thank you, Phoebe, for having been such a wonderful teacher.

John M. Fink
Santa Barbara, California

Introduction

Third Opinion is strictly an information resource. Most of the programs detailed here are nutritional, metabolic, "immune enhancing," biological, or behavioral-psychological. Besides alternative therapy (given instead of conventional treatment) and adjunctive therapy (given with conventional treatment), they are often called complementary, unconventional, unorthodox, and nontoxic treatments. They are referred to by the American Cancer Society as unproven, although it has been pointed out that this is not the same as disproven. Many are considered holistic; they treat the whole body. They are relatively nontoxic—nondestructive to healthy cells. They often heal the body on many levels—mental, emotional, and spiritual, as well as physical. They often rely on a variety of substances, as opposed to a single substance, to stimulate the immune system and promote healing. (These multiple variables are one reason that current scientific standards are so hard to apply to these methods.) Moreover, these programs are usually aimed toward the cause of the disease and not just the symptoms.

The entire field of alternatives is vast and encompasses territory ranging from prayer to electromagnetic treatment. Although some may not be represented here, this book covers the majority of the better-known alternative therapies.

Doctors vary in their approaches to cancer. Patients commonly get second opinions, even several "second" opinions. However, rarely, especially in the United States, will a conventional doctor give you an enlightened opinion about nutrition and other nontoxic alternatives. For this reason, as well as the fact that there has been so little progress in healing the major cancers and other degenerative diseases, the interest in alternatives runs very high.

Although *Third Opinion* isn't for everyone, it may be for those who haven't found help in conventional treatments and are still looking and hoping. It could be for those who aren't ready to accept an "expert's" word as the final judgment ("you only have six months to a year to live"). It may also be for those people who want to assume responsibility for their own treatments, for those who are concerned about the quality of their lives, and for those who are looking for a gentler approach to healing in cancer, heart disease, arthritis, diabetes, multiple sclerosis, lupus, AIDS, or other degenerative diseases. And it could be for some of those patients who want to complement their conventional treatments or reduce or eliminate the toxic side effects of those treatments.

Of course, this guide can and should serve those who are looking for ways to prevent the occurrence of cancer and other degenerative diseases. The diet-based programs are usually geared toward prevention. The importance of prevention cannot be overemphasized. Following the lead of the National Academy of Sciences' historic 1982 report *Diet, Nutrition, and Cancer,* we can all begin by following the National Cancer Institute's and American Cancer Society's dietary recommendations regarding fat reduction along with an increase of fiber, including fresh fruits, vegetables, and whole-grain breads and cereals. At the very least, we should be moderate with potentially addictive substances such as alcohol, caffeine, sugar, and sodium. And it should go without saying that we should stop smoking and limit our exposure to environmental carcinogens: toxic substances and pollution. To all of this, add regular exercise. Among the material here is much that can be useful in the field of prevention, for ourselves and future generations.

I hope this book lists all of the nitty-gritty information about clinics, doctors, health practitioners, educators, support groups, and research and information organizations. Because the field is so vast, it would take another book to present an in-depth description and discussion of the therapies, underlying philosophies, supportive studies, case studies, and testimonials. For the same reason, I don't explore the historical, political, or sociological aspects of alternatives. That kind of information can be gathered from the many books and articles listed in the bibliography and under the various entries.

This book begins with guidelines that should be kept in mind as you consider the various programs under discussion. The bulk of the book is divided into four sections: Treatment Centers, which includes places where people can go for programs; Educational Centers, which lists places where people can be educated about programs, including some research institutes; Support Groups, which details programs giving behavioral-psychological support, imagery training, and, in a few cases, material support; and Information Services, which explores organizations that specialize in information about all or some of the above and which lists patients' organizations as well.

As many approaches are somewhat eclectic, there is a certain amount of overlap in some of these categories. Every section should be read to make sure that nothing of value was skipped. To make it easier for readers to find resources in a certain geographical area, a region-by-region listing has been provided. Also included is a glossary of terms and abbreviations, and a bibliography. Telephone numbers given throughout this book have been coded, whenever possible, to facilitate direct dialing from the United States.

For some people, some of these methods may prove very difficult, both emotionally and physically. The support of family, friends, and other helpers is very important. It has been suggested that stress can slow down or even stop the healing process, so if the necessary support isn't there or if something is contrary to your belief system, it might be better to find a therapy you can participate in willingly and positively. Also, I fully support a person's choice to let go of the fight to survive whenever he or she feels that time has come.

It has been my dream over these past years to help bridge the gap between the worlds of conventional and alternative medicine. I believe that a patient is entitled to make an informed choice based on all the available information, and it is with this belief that I write this book. I urge you to keep an open mind about all therapies, whether they are conventional or unconventional. Each situation dictates a unique response. And I hope that considering these programs will not stop you from looking at conventional approaches, to use either alone or adjunctively, and pursuing them if they seem the most appropriate. Conventional programs, even the experimental ones, should be much easier to gather information about than those that follow, the difference being that conventional programs are sanctioned by the medical community while these are not.

Because the United States, unlike so many other countries, supports only one kind of medicine, Americans have overlooked many aspects of the art of healing. Economic, political, and professional pressures on institutional medicine have helped create an environment that deters the exploration of new avenues of research. This has made it very difficult for the health professionals outside of orthodox medicine to practice. It has also made it difficult for medical doctors to incorporate lesser-known healing methods into their practice. Because so many of them have been legislated against, harassed, prosecuted, and discredited, it is a wonder that so many of the champions of these therapies have managed to keep their programs available.

I must say a word here about quackery, as this, unfortunately, comes up so often. According to the late Congressman Claude Pepper's 1984 hearings on quackery, a quack is "anyone who promotes medical schemes or remedies known to be false, or which are unproven, for a profit." Now, of course, there are quacks out there who will try to take advantage of a cancer patient's situation for profit, both outside and inside mainstream medicine. And deceit, pretense, and fraud in serious medical matters are inexcusable and criminal. But it seems unfair to categorize unorthodox healing methods as quackery simply because they are "unproven." A United States government report* states, "it has been estimated that only 10%–20% of all procedures currently used in medical practice have been shown to be efficacious by controlled trial." By this definition, wouldn't that make the remaining 80%–90% of accepted medical procedures in the United States quackery?

I have seen many ethical practitioners using these therapies, helping people, working under duress, documenting their cases, and trying to get their programs recognized. It's a shame that these practitioners can't get the attention of established medicine and receive funding for their research.

Some United States congressmen took a step in the right direction when they requested the congressional Office of Technology Assessment do a comprehensive report on *Unconventional Cancer Treatments*. This first government-sponsored look into these therapies, published in September 1990, cites many of the positive studies supporting these

---

*Assessing the Efficacy and Safety of Medical Technologies, PB 286/929, Office of Technology Assessment, September 1978.

therapies while acknowledging the failure of orthodox treatments to make much more than minimal progress in bringing most cancers under control.

The report mentions the growing number of medical practitioners who choose to combine what they feel is the best of both alternative and conventional treatments, as well as noting how difficult it is to use unconventional methods in today's medical/legal climate. Stating that some of these methods may be adopted by mainstream practice in the years ahead, the report refers to recent progress in the psycho-social field, with the comment that many feel the next breakthroughs will occur in the nutritional area. It suggests the National Cancer Institute could take a more active part regarding unconventional treatments, such as by providing funds for conducting evaluations.

I continue to look forward to the day when these therapies can be fairly assessed. In the meantime, before you undertake a program, the best means of precaution is to talk to people who've used it. The many patients who attribute their recoveries to alternative therapies will serve as a valuable source of help, inspiration, and information. Ask to talk to patients. Strong recommendations are a good defense against quackery.

You, the consumer, must be aware that there are people out there who will try to take advantage of your situation. The responsibility is yours to determine, through diligent research, who those people are, and then to avoid them. It is a fact that not everyone who tries a therapy, any therapy, is helped by it. It is also a fact that bad as well as good experiences occur with any therapy. To a large degree, your success will depend on when you go, who you see, and what you bring to that experience. Your attitude may be the factor that tips the scale toward good wherever you go.

Information can come to you in many ways, but you can't necessarily rely on an alternative doctor—just as you can't necessarily rely on an orthodox doctor—for all the information you may require. You are really on a solitary journey, and you should be encouraged to participate actively in your own recovery and perform your own research.

Everyone listed here was contacted by us and responded to our questions. If you cannot find a listing of the people or centers in which you're interested, we apologize. In a few cases, people have asked not to be included, perhaps to avoid the kind of harassment often faced by professionals in this field. In some special cases, we decided that the reputation of a place was not good enough to justify its inclusion. However, it could be that we simply haven't heard of certain programs. If you will, send their names and addresses to Third Opinion, P.O. Box 50114, Santa Barbara, California 93150. We will get in touch with them before the next update.

There is a questionnaire for patients' comments in the very back of the book. Any feedback you can give us about your experience will be very useful and greatly appreciated. Just remove the questionnaire from the book, fill it in, and send it to the address on the form.

This book is an ongoing project. Since information becomes outdated as time passes, both the publisher and I are updating, revising, and reprinting *Third Opinion* to make it even more comprehensive.

I have not visited all the places listed in this directory, nor have I met all the practitioners. Although I have been involved with the International Association of Cancer Victors and Friends and with the National Health Federation, both information organizations, and have spoken before on this subject, it should not be construed that I am promoting or advocating any therapies or making recommendations of any kind. Nor should it be thought that I am assuming any responsibility for the decisions you may make. I am a layman passing on information for the reader to evaluate. A knowledgeable physician should be consulted regarding the medical aspects of any therapy.

It is my greatest hope that you will enjoy your search, that you will find what you need, and that your health will improve as a result of your efforts.

John Fink's Testimony Before the U.S. Senate Committee on Labor and Human Resources Hearing on "Nutrition and Fitness," Chaired by Senator Orrin Hatch, with Senator Edward Kennedy, Ranking Minority Member, November 13, 1985

I had been an actor for fourteen years when eight years ago, my two-year-old daughter was diagnosed as having a rare form of cancer. When doctors told us her prognosis was not good, my wife and I did what many loving parents do: we looked at anything and everything that could possibly help her. Our daughter lived only two years longer, but we feel that the quality of her short life was enhanced by the use of complementary treatments.

During our search we were surprised to find that many people with cancer were staying alive and well using natural methods. Some had advanced cancers and had been told by their doctors to go home and get their affairs in order. Many of these people are still alive today. This discovery consumed us.

For the past five years my wife and I have helped hold together a group in Santa Barbara called the Cancer Victors. Made up of around one hundred members, this group includes people with cancer, their families, and their friends. Those who have cancer are controlling it with nontoxic, primarily nutritional methods used exclusively or in conjunction with conventional treatments. Our work is volunteered and fills most of our time.

In 1982 I took several trips with professional researchers* visiting major hospitals, clinics, and physicians throughout the United States, Europe, and Mexico. During this trip I explored various complementary therapies and investigated the newest avenues of health research, prevention, and treatment of cancer and other degenerative diseases.

I have brought two articles by Dr. Michael Lerner, one of the researchers. Published in *Advances*, the journal of the Institute for the Advancement of

---

*Michael Lerner, PhD, who is a MacArthur Prize Fellow at the Institute for Health Policy Studies, University of California San Francisco School of Medicine. He is president and founder of Commonweal, a center for research in health and human ecology in Bolinas, California. Also, Dr. Sandra McLanahan, M.D., who is a physician from Charlottesville and Buckingham, Virginia.

Health, these articles detail our findings and make them available for anyone interested.

In short, although we found no silver bullet cures, we found people who were reversing or at least holding their cancers in remission through the use of these therapies. As one example, we were very impressed with the Bristol Cancer Help Centre in England, officially opened by Prince Charles. The centre's program emphasizes a change of lifestyle, nutrition, and stress control, which often are added to conventional treatments to enhance the patients' response and powers of self-healing.

It made me sad to read Harvard statistician John Cairns' article, published in the November 1985 issue of *Scientific American*, in which Cairns said that of the more than 200,000 American patients receiving chemotherapy, the number of patients being cured could not exceed more than a few percent.

As Prince Charles said while addressing the British Medical Association: "It is frightening how dependent upon drugs we are all becoming and how easy it is for doctors to prescribe them as the universal panacea for all ills. Wonderful as many of them are, it should still be more widely stressed by doctors that the health of human beings is so often determined by their behaviour, their food, and the nature of their environment."

In our group in Santa Barbara, we see cancer patients coming back month after month who are keeping their cancer in remission by themselves using natural means. Many of them are aged. It often requires enormous determination, will, and courage to follow a rigid diet and do it alone, and their remissions seem anything but "spontaneous." What is tragic is that some of these people have to leave this country to find doctors who will or can monitor and support their progress while using these therapies.

I support groups such as the International Association of Cancer Victors and Friends and the National Health Federation* because, among other reasons, they are two of the few organizations supplying this difficult-to-get information about where people can go to find, for example, metabolic therapies, diet therapies, immune therapies, botanical therapies, and help in mental imagery. But this is not enough.

It is time that every doctor in this country recognizes the importance of nutrition and the mind, not only in preventing disease, but in helping to overcome disease. There is now a wealth of scientific information establishing the link between nutrition and the cause of some major forms of cancer. Clinical

---

*These organizations were mentioned because of my association with them at the time. Please see information services for a complete listing.

practice is showing us that nutrition can be an important complementary therapy.

Congress is to be commended for encouraging in the seventies the National Cancer Institute to set up the Diet, Nutrition, and Cancer Program, and for the creation of the Dietary Goals Report. Now the Congress, you Senators, can further the cause of improved health by calling for new research using nutrition in the treatment of cancer.

Thank you.

This study shows that many patients receiving alternative care do not conform to the traditional stereotype of poorly educated, terminally ill patients who have exhausted conventional treatment. Similarly, although some unorthodox practitioners may well fit the characteristic portrait of quacks and charlatans, many are well-trained, few charge high fees, and most, on the basis of patients' views and our own observations, sincerely believe in the efficacy and rationality of their work. Contemporary alternatives, unlike the pills and potions of the past, are long-term, lifestyle-oriented options that exist within a broad view of health and personal responsibility. Patients welcome the self-care role and the concomitant responsibility to attain health. . . . The emphasis of unorthodox therapy on nutrition, health as a personal responsibility, pollution, and purification has religious and moral overtones, but also represents themes of great importance not only to patients, but to science and society as well. As such, unorthodox therapy is unlikely to be readily discarded.

> *"Contemporary Unorthodox*
> *Treatments in Cancer Medicine"*
> *Barrie Cassileth, Ph.D. et al.*
> Annals of Internal Medicine
> July 1984

Half of the people interviewed said that clinics that treat cancer and other degenerative diseases in ways opposed by the established medical community should be allowed to operate in the United States.

> *Associated Press—Media General Poll*
> *September 1–7, 1985*

Guidelines for Choosing
a Therapy

The guidelines that follow should help in narrowing the choices presented here. Making decisions can be difficult. Even though the differences among the programs may be confusing, each one does not postulate a brand new principle. Look for the unity in the common underlying principles that are a part of so many of these approaches; they are often variations on the same theme. It helps to understand the concepts involved; if you don't already understand them, further reading may be essential. Examine each program carefully, but see it as a potential opportunity for getting well. Many of these guidelines can be applied to any therapy, whether mentioned in this book or not.

Similarities

A common denominator of many of the therapies is the idea that the body should rebuild itself through the use of fine nutrition, vitamins, minerals, and/or other "immune stimulators" that work as keys to activate the healing process. Some therapies emphasize that the body should first be detoxified through a cleansing process. Many of these theories are distantly related to the field of orthodox immunology but differ from most conventional treatments, which specifically target cancer cells but in the process can damage much more in the human organism.

These methods often deal with relatively harmless substances on the physical level, attitudinal changes on the psychological level, and the acknowledgment of some greater force on the spiritual level. They often are said to treat the cause, not just the symptoms.

Free Time

The more of this you have, the more options you may have. If you have to work full time, some treatments will be too time consuming for you. Others, though, may be compatible with a busy schedule once you've begun. Some therapies are almost impossible to do without devoting your full time to them, at least initially. It is very important to recognize your limitations so that you don't commit to something unless you are in a position to follow through on it.

Belief Systems

If a particular therapy has some aspects that are going to add more stress to your life and you aren't able to curb your resistance, it may be best to look elsewhere. For example, I've seen a strict diet that is acceptable to one person be intolerable to another. (It's difficult to maintain belief in something you can't stomach.) Some programs built on a foundation of strong religious beliefs might not be suitable for someone who doesn't share those beliefs. I've seen meditation, as part of a program, conflict with a patient's religious convictions. There is a growing awareness that it makes a difference in what you have faith in, whether your faith is conscious or unconscious.

Comparisons and Statistics

Try to get information about people who have had a related cancer. Some information organizations, and some clinics as well, have lists of recovered patients who you can talk to. Call or write to these people, if you can, and ask what they specifically did that has helped them. Compare with conventional therapy results. These may be the most important questions you pursue, so spend some time on this.

With limited resources—no time, energy, or money—many alternative therapists find it impossible to compile statistics that would be acceptable to established medicine. And most of them simply don't have the capacity to do proper follow-ups. Again, you can ask for successful case studies. Unfortunately, statistics are questionable across the board— John Bailar of Harvard, in a 1986 study in the *New England Journal of Medicine*, and the Government's 1987 General Accounting Office report both questioned the inflated conventional survival statistics stated by the National Cancer Institute.

Caveat emptor: Some doctors and clinics seem to be fond of concocting their own questionably high response and cure rates. Find out exactly what is meant by "response." Regard all cure and remission rates with some caution, and ask for documented cases and testimonials from clinics and doctors; sometimes you can get them.

Distance

A trip to another country might prove challenging and exotic to one person and debilitating to another. Language differences can be an obstacle, and clinics in other countries may not live up to what you have come to expect at home. Of course, they also may be just the tonic for you.

If you are unable for some reason to get to a center, then remember that some people have successfully undertaken programs at home.

Finances

You don't need the added stress of committing yourself to something that is financially over your head. There is a wide range of treatment costs, so think it through ahead of time. Take care to compare prices. You can do this most easily with centers that offer almost identical programs. Even though some prices may be outdated by the time you read this, if you consider the rough time frame in which they're current, they should form a good base for comparison. All prices are subject to change without notification, so check to confirm. Some programs will allow you to pay what you can afford. As many of these programs don't advertise this policy, you will need to ask specific questions.

Some therapies are covered by some insurance. This is a tricky area and always changing, so it's hard to give any hard-and-fast rules about how to handle this. Keep asking and trying.

Physical Condition

Your capacity for self-care and the extent of your illness will have a lot to do with your choice. Many therapies will take a lot of energy and might be next to impossible for some patients to accomplish on their own. For instance, getting supplies in bulk, growing certain foods, preparing particular diets and juices, and performing special procedures often require assistance. Sad to report, there is little active cooperation among the clinics, which means that if you end up in a program that isn't working for you and you want to try a different program, you should not expect to be referred elsewhere. You will need emotional and physical reserves to accomplish the move.

Clarity

Before you go to a clinic or an alternative practitioner, try to pin down exactly what you'll be getting and at what cost. That way you may avoid unwelcome surprises. Ask about patients you can talk to, find out about the length of stay and what you need to bring. Pin down what a practitioner means by "response" (get details on long- or short-term survival and ask questions about quality of life: lack of side effects, reduced or eliminated pain, enhanced well-being, etc.).

Some therapies have supportive studies to back them up; if not published in the United States, they are sometimes published in other countries. You can request to see them.

If you are going to another country and think there could be any confusion at all regarding arrangements, don't be afraid to check and recheck before you go.

Adjunctive Therapy

If it's important to you, when you contact a place ask whether the program can be used adjunctively as well as alternatively. The coordination of conventional and unconventional treatments could be crucial, so don't do this without good professional guidance. For example, if you are following a special diet on your own, be aware that it may not be compatible with chemotherapy. It's best to ask the right questions first.

Best Responders

If you are attracted to a center because of the responses you read under the listings, remember that these claims may be unverified; request that a place back up its claims by citing cases that you can verify. Some places did not specify which cancers have been most successfully treated by their program. Try to narrow it down to a type of cancer by specifying the cell type and stage of the cancer. If a place does not list a specific cancer, you should not assume that they are not having results with that type of cancer.

Be aware that all mentions of acquired immune deficiency syndrome (AIDS) are in response to a specific question we asked; we have no information to support the results.

Support

This is an extremely important area to consider; not only will the emotional support of your family and friends be important, but you may also need the physical support of someone to help you with the program. If support doesn't exist among those close to you, you may want to find people who are sympathetic and supportive. Support group and information resource listings should be of great value in this area.

Verification and Consultation

This comprehensive list of people and places should in no way be understood to mean that either the author or the publisher recommends or endorses any of these therapies. The information was derived from questionnaires that were sent out and returned, along with other materials, and we did not make personal investigations into the accuracy of all the claims made here. Every patient should make his or her own investigation of the information on the list. In addition, it would be wise to consult with a knowledgeable physician before undertaking a therapy. Try to find a doctor who is sympathetic to your point of view. Obviously, this may take some time, but it will be worth the effort. A physician who listens with an open mind can be an invaluable source of support and guidance.

AFTER YOU CHOOSE A THERAPY

When you make a choice, do your very best to follow through. If you are bothered by the disorganization and confusion you might find at some centers, try to remain open and to give the program a fair trial. Do not abandon the program for reasons that may simply be conditioned prejudice. Beyond the surface, there may be much merit.

As with any therapy, close observation is important. Be alert to progress being made. Stay open to trying something different if what you're doing clearly isn't working or is working against you. Augmenting some therapies with parts of others may be okay, and by asking, you may find out about other people who have done this successfully; it may work for you, too. However, everyone is biochemically unique, so one person's needs may be different from another's.

The importance of your attitude cannot be overemphasized. Being confused over any period of time can only add to stress and may therefore impede the healing process. As mentioned earlier, when examining these choices, look for the unifying principle underlying most of them. See these choices as possibilities, opportunities, and gifts—which is what they are—and not as additional burdens. Believe it or not, I have often heard people say that getting cancer was the best thing that ever happened to them. By that they meant that with their backs to the wall, they finally found the motivation to examine and change their lifestyles and develop a strong will to live. On the subject of false hope, they say that there is no such thing.

Treatment Centers

Hospitals, Clinics, Physicians, Health Practitioners
North America (Bahamas, Canada, Mexico, United States)

Akbar Clinic

(Panama City Clinic)
236 South Tyndall Parkway
Panama City, Florida 32404
United States

(904) 763–7689
Fax: (904) 763–5396

Primary Personnel

Ahmed Elkadi, M.D., administrator.

Directions

The clinic is located in northwestern Florida in Panama City at the Wal-Mart shopping center, behind Captain D's restaurant in Parker.

Background

The Akbar Clinic was established in June 1984. It offers all conventional medical, surgical, pediatric, dental, and counseling services in addition to the multimodality immunotherapy program, which is a unique, comprehensive nontoxic metabolic therapy designed to enhance or restore the body's immune system. The protocol is based in part on the work of Dr. Josef Issels. It is useful in the treatment of conditions associated with immune deficiency. A multispecialty ambulatory medical facility is housed in a 6,000-square-foot, two-story building. Arrangements can be made for any number of patients. Five languages are spoken there: English, French, Spanish, German, and Arabic.

Illness Treated

All illnesses, including cancer, AIDS, and chronic degenerative diseases. They've reported good responses in patients with a variety of far advanced metastatic cancers, including those with cancer of the breast, colon, pancreas, throat, and others.

Treatment Offered

The multimodality immunotherapy program is a nontoxic metabolic treatment with virtually no side effects. It includes nutritional adjustment; nutritional supplementation with certain vitamins, minerals, and enzymes; several natural immune enhancers; acupuncture; hyperpyrexia (fever therapy); infusion with vitamins, chelation, HCl, and ozone; biofeedback; counseling; exercise; and removing any focus of chronic infections. The clinic is undertaking a clinical trial of the program.

Related Readings

Immunotherapy in Progressive Metastatic Cancer by J. Issels, M.D.

Effect of Nigella Sativa (The Black Seed) and Immunity by A. Elkadi, M.D., and O. Kandil.

The Black Seed (Nigella Sativa) and Immunity by A. Elkadi, M.D., and O. Kandil.

The clinic will also provide upon request information regarding past patients.

Length of Treatment/Stay

Patients in the multimodality immunotherapy program require an average of two months. A home maintenance program is also available.

Costs

$1,500 to $2,200 a week includes physician's fee, counseling, biofeedback, physical therapy, acupuncture, intravenous drip with medication, hyperpyrexia medication taken by mouth, blood and urine tests, immune studies, chest X-ray, and EKG. Additional studies that may be needed according to the nature of the disease are extra. Room and board is also extra.

Method of Payment

Cash, traveler's checks, bank drafts, American Express, Visa, MasterCard, private insurance, Medicare, Medicaid, and Workmen's Compensation are accepted.

Alternative Health Center

1744 Highway 95, Suite 12
Bullhead City, Arizona 86442
United States

(602) 758–8899
(702) 298–8043
(800) 446–7548

Contact Person

Glenda.

Primary Personnel

Michael Vonk, D.N.

Directions

Take highway I-40 to I-95 leading to Bullhead City.

Background

Dr. Vonk has studied in Japan, China, and Europe. He has a strong background in herbs, Chinese medicine, and nutrition.

Illness Treated

All cancers, AIDS, and arthritis. The center also treats the spectre of chronic degenerative health problems, such as cariovascular problems.

Treatment Offered

An interdisciplinary approach through herbs, nutrition counseling, lifestyle assessment, stress management, and control of habits. The clinic offers Kanpoyaku, an Oriental herbal treatment for the specific management of cancers. The patient should first send information regarding the particular illness, then contact the center to make necessary arrangements. All treatments are on an outpatient basis.

Related Readings

East/West Cancer Remedies for Wellness & Recovery by Hye Koo Yun.

Length of Treatment/Stay

Oral chelation requires a one-day stay at the center. Cancer, AIDS, and arthritis patients would need three days at the center, although the treatment would continue for months at home.

Costs

Motel: $90 (average).
Cancer, AIDS: $4,975 for three months of treatment.
Arthritis: $2,600–$5,000 for six months to a year.
Oral chelation (for cardiovascular problems): $625 for six weeks.
Additional treatment such as enzymes, minerals, or personalized care would cost extra.

Method of Payment

The clinic asks that the patient pay in full the first day. Personal checks are accepted, but money orders or traveler's checks are preferred. Visa and MasterCard are also accepted. Insurance is accepted, but be sure to check with your insurance company first.

American Biologics-
Mexico S.A. Medical Center

United States Admissions Office:
1180 Walnut Avenue
Chula Vista, California 92011
United States

(619) 429–8200
(800) 227–4458
(800) 227–4473

Clinic:
#15 Azucenas Street
Tijuana, B.C.
Mexico

Contact Person

Michael L. Culbert, D. Sc.

Primary Personnel

Rodrigo Rodriguez, M.D., medical director; Wolfram Kuhnau, M.D.; Robert Bradford, Ph.D. (Hon.).

Directions

The clinic is located off Agua Caliente Boulevard.

Background

American Biologics-Mexico S.A. Medical Center, located in Tijuana, Mexico, is 35 minutes from the San Diego airport. This clinic has inpatient and outpatient care facilities. It offers a complete diagnostic laboratory screening, which includes standardized blood analysis, HLB and LBA blood monitoring, X-rays, CAT scan, and access, if necessary, to complete cobalt and other facilities. Standard orthodox therapies are available and integrated when jointly agreed upon by the medical staff and patient. Modern private and semiprivate rooms are available.

Illness Treated

Cancer and other degenerative illnesses.

Treatment Offered

Eclectic, metabolic, nutrition, ACN bioelectricity, live cell therapy, tumor liquefaction, tumor blockers, butyrate complex and staphage-lysate in lymph system connected cancer, aqueous solutions of injectable laetrile, megavitamins/minerals, herbal nonsurgical tumor removal, enzyme treatments, hydrazine sulfate, chondroitin sulfate, DMSO therapy, gerovital, experimental vaccines and biologicals, therapeutic nutrition tailored for the individual, sophisticated adjunctive therapies, EDTA chelation therapy (intravenous and oral), gastro-intestinal tract cleansing, and detoxification.

Related Readings

Cancer Protocols by Robert Bradford and Michael Culbert.

Metabolic Management of Cancer by Robert Bradford and Michael Culbert.

Choice Magazine, sponsored by the Committee for Freedom of Choice in Medicine Inc.

What the Medical Establishment Won't Tell You That Could Save Your Life by Michael Culbert. 1983.

Now That You Have Cancer by Robert Bradford and Michael Culbert. 1984.

Oxidology: The Study of Reactive Oxygen Toxic Species (ROTS) *and Their Metabolism in Health and Disease* by Robert Bradford, Michael Culbert, and Henry W. Allen.

The Biochemical Basis of Live-Cell Therapy by Robert Bradford, Michael Culbert, and Henry W. Allen.

AIDS: Hope—Hoax—Hoopla by Michael Culbert.

Length of Treatment/Stay

Five days to three weeks.

Costs

Live cell therapy costs $2,700 for five days of treatment, including hotel. A 10-day total program costs $4,300. Live cell therapy injections alone are $200 per dosage. Degenerative conditions such as cancer, lupus, multiple sclerosis, emphysema, and others cost $1,900 for the first week and $1,700 for each additional week as an outpatient or $3,000 for each week of hospitalization. A consultation visit may be arranged for $50. A diagnostic workup/consultation without treatment is $500. There is a recommended support program for patients at an additional cost.

Method of Payment

Most American insurance companies reimburse patients. Traveler's checks, certified checks, money orders, Visa, MasterCard, and American Express are accepted. No personal checks are accepted.

American Metabolic Institute

(Hospital Metabolic G. Rubio-Fry)

Mailing Address:
524 Calle Primera Road, Suite 1005A
San Ysidro, California 92173
United States

(619) 229–3003
(619) 662–1082
011 52 66 13–12–40
011 52 66 13–13–40
(800) 388–1083
(706) 613–1240

Clinic:
La Gloria area between Tijuana and Rosarito Beach, Mexico.

Primary Personnel

Geronimo Rubio, M.D. medical director; William R. Fry, marketing director; Kenneth Johnson, D.C., N.D., physiotherapy director.

Directions

La Gloria is on Highway 1, the old road to Rosarito Ensenada out of Tijuana.

Background

The inpatient clinic is seven years old. It specializes in treating cancer and degenerative diseases. Diagnostic tests include: blood crystalization test, live cell analysis, iridology, kinesiology, traditional physicals, SMAC, CEA, CBC, urine, sonagram, CAT scan, and X-ray.

Illness Treated

Cancer and degenerative diseases.

Treatment Offered

Herbal salves on melanoma, detoxification programs (fasting, colonic, sweat baths), bioelectrical medicine, hydrogen peroxide, laetrile, lymphatic massage, reflexology, clay baths, ultrasound, acupressure, hydrotherapy, chelation, live cell therapy, immunology vitamins, amino acids, digestive enzymes, herbs, homeopathic remedies, vegetarian nutrition program, color therapy, magnet therapy, music therapy, ozone therapy, hyperbaric oxygen (HBO) therapy, attitudinal work, and classes.

Length of Treatment/Stay

Private rooms with bath, shower, and television are provided for all patients and their support person. Programs run between two and four weeks, or longer. Treatment continues at home for one year, with monitoring done by the clinic.

Costs

Cancer program: $7,400 for three weeks.
Candida program: $4,900 for two weeks.
Detoxification program: $4,200 for two weeks.
Detoxification program: $1,700 for one week.
Added weeks: $1,950 per week.
Companions: $35 per day.

Method of Payment

Cashier's checks, credit cards, traveler's checks, and cash are accepted upon admission. Call ahead with credit card information for verification. To check on insurance coverage, call (713) 953–0906.

Atkins Center for Complementary Medicine

152 East 55th Street
New York, New York 10022
United States

(212) 758–2110
Fax: (212) 754–4284

Contact Person

New patient representatives are Jane, Rene, and Gazlea.

Primary Personnel

Robert C. Atkins, M.D.; Stuart Fischer, M.D.; and Nancy Hancock, administrator.

Directions

Located in midtown Manhattan, accessible by public transportation.

Background

Dr. Atkins has been in the forefront of the nutrition medicine movement ever since the publication of his book *Dr. Atkins' Diet Revolution.* He graduated from Cornell University Medical College, trained in cardiology, is president of the Foundation for the Advancement of Innovative Medicine, and is a member of the American College of Advancement in Medicine. He hosts "Design for Living," the longest-running health-related radio program in the United States.

Illness Treated

Cancer of all types, with especially favorable results for prostate and lung cancer. Also treats blood sugar disorders, chronic fatigue syndrome, autoimmune disorders, cardiovascular diseases, allergies, asthma, obesity, disturbances of lipid metabolism, and other chronic illnesses. The center prefers patients who have no prior exposure to chemotherapy or radiation.

Treatment Offered

Nutritionally based treatments, including oral vitamin and mineral therapy, dietary regulation, and an intensive intravenous program. Modalities include integrated protocols with herbal therapies, germanium, pancreatic enzymes, and oxygenating therapies.

Related Readings

Dr. Atkins' Health Revolution by Robert C. Atkins, M.D.

Dr. Atkins' Superenergy Diet by Robert C. Atkins, M.D.

Dr. Atkins' Nutrition Breakthrough by Robert C. Atkins, M.D.

Dr. Atkins' Diet Revolution by Robert C. Atkins, M.D.

Length of Treatment/Stay

Intensive intravenous therapy requires frequent and periodic re-evaluations of blood parameters, of physical findings, and of standard procedures such as sonography, gastro-intestinal scans, etc. But there are no inpatient facilities; patients must make their own arrangements for housing.

Costs

Varies, depending on the type and extent of the illness and on the patient's response to treatment. An initial evaluation, on the average, costs $350–$600. Additional costs—such as follow-up office visits, periodic laboratory evaluations, oral vitamin and mineral program, and intravenous therapy—not submitted for publication.

Paul Beals, M.D.

9101 Cherry Lane, Suite 205
Laurel, Maryland 20708
United States

(301) 490–9911

2639 Connecticut Avenue N.W.
Suite 100C
Washington, D.C. 20008
United States

(202) 332–0370

Office Hours
In Maryland: Monday–Thursday, 8:30 a.m.–12:00 p.m.;
Monday, Wednesday, 2:30–4:30 p.m.; Tuesday, Thursday, 2:30–7:00 p.m.;
Saturday, 8:30 a.m.–12:00 p. m.
In Washington D.C.: Friday, 9 a.m.–1 p.m.

Primary Personnel

Paul Beals, M.D.

Directions

Washington D.C. Beltway (95) to Baltimore Washington Parkway to 197 north to Cherry
Lane (left turn).

Background

Dr. Beals is heard regularly on the local Baltimore television and radio stations. He treats
patients who have degenerative disorders. He treats the physical, mental, emotional, and
spiritual nature of a patient. He is board certified in family practice. Dr. Beals is a member of
the American Academy of Family Physicians and the American College of Advancement in
Medicine.

Illness Treated

Most nonmetastatic cancers, arthritis, heart disease, vascular disease, and Alzheimer's
disease.

Treatment Offered

Nutritional, metabolic, immunotherapy, laetrile, megavitamins, and hair analysis. Patients are put on a nutritional program and given vitamins, minerals, enzymes, and nontoxic vaccines to help build up the immune system. There are no toxic or significant side effects except for nausea.

Related Readings

The Death of Cancer by Harold W. Manner. Advanced Century Publishing, 1978.

The Cancer Survivors and How They Did It by Judith Glassman. Dial Press, 1983.

The clinic will also furnish upon request information regarding past patients.

Length of Treatment/Stay

Three to six months for outpatient therapies.

Costs

$400 to $700 a month.

Method of Payment

Payment is required at the time of visit. Cash, personal checks, MasterCard, and Visa are all accepted. Submit itemized bill to your insurance company for reimbursement, but check with them first. Blue Shield and Medicare participate in this program as well.

Bio-Medical Center

P.O. Box 727
General Ferreira #615
Colonia Juarez
Tijuana, B.C.
Mexico

011–52–66–84–90–11
          84–90–81
          84–90–82
          84–93–76
Fax: 011–52–66–84–97–44

Primary Personnel

Fernando Arriola, M.D.; Mildred Nelson, R.N.

Directions

Patients can stay at E-Z8 Motel (619) 223–9500 in San Diego and call for transportation at (619) 226–8655 with Leona Rogers or stay at International Motor Inn (619) 428–4486 in San Ysidro. They have a free shuttle bus to the clinic.

Background

The Hoxsey therapy was started in 1840, when it was used on a horse with a cancerous sore on its leg. This formula was passed down through the Hoxsey family and has been used internally and externally on humans for more than 50 years. Mildred Nelson, R.N., now operates this clinic, which has been in Tijuana since 1963 and formerly was run by the late Harry Hoxsey.

This is an outpatient clinic only. Appointments usually last one full day, sometimes up to three days, with a follow-up visit three to six months later, if possible. Patients are requested to arrive by 8:30 a.m. without having eaten breakfast and having taken a laxative the night before. Patents are given a complete workup in the morning, and meet with the doctors in the afternoon. Appointments are not necessary. (But the clinic is closed on all legal holidays of the United States; on five Mexican holidays—February 5, March 21, May 1, September 16, and November 20; and for the last two weeks of December.)

Illness Treated

Cancer; the best responders are lymphoma, melanoma, and external (skin). Also Candida albicans and Epstein Barr virus syndrome.

Treatment Offered

Hoxsey treatment, vitamins, diet, immune stimulation, and Candida treatment. The Hoxsey formula is a liquid tonic made from potassium iodide and the following herbs: licorice, red clover, cascara, burdock root, barberis root, poke root, and stillingia root; it is used for internal cancers. There is also a salve and a powder used on external cancers. The patients take the prescribed tonic or salve and nutritional supplements; follow some diet specifications, such as no tomatoes, vinegar, pork, or alcohol; and are asked to avoid salt, sugar, and white flour products.

Related Readings

You Don't Have to Die by Harry M. Hoxsey. Joseph C. Carl, 1977.

Hoxsey Quacks Who Cure Cancer (a film). Realidad Productions.

Length of Treatment/Stay

One to three days.

Costs

The treatment, which includes office calls, doctors' fees, and medications for as long as necessary (for life), costs $3,500. On the first visit, 30% of cost must be paid; the rest will be arranged in monthly payments. X-ray, laboratory, and physical charges run from $450 to $850. Currently, all patients are tested first for Candida albicans.

Method of Payment

Personal checks, traveler's checks, and cash in United States funds are accepted. No credit cards are accepted.

Brian E. Briggs, M.D.

718 6th Street S.W.
Minot, North Dakota 58701
United States

(701) 838–6011

Contact Person

Dr. Briggs or secretary.

Primary Personnel

Brian E. Briggs, M.D.

Directions

Broadway to 11th Avenue S.W.; then four blocks west to 6th Street S.W.; then approximately four blocks north.

Background

Dr. Briggs is a 1954 graduate of the University of Minnesota (M.D.). He had orthodox experience (medicine and surgery) before beginning holistic training and practice. The primary focus is on causative stress and environmental elements. The center takes three new patients per day and has twelve chelators.

Illness Treated

Cancer; the best responder is prostate. Also cardiovascular disorders, immune system disorders, and psychological and chemical disorders.

Treatment Offered

Detoxification, elimination of environmental poisons, neural therapy, nutritional counseling, prescription drugs, and intravenous therapy of chelation and vitamins (with additional amygdalin in cancer patients).

Related Readings

Get Well—Stay Well (booklet for new patients). 1984.

Length of Treatment/Stay

One day to two weeks.

Costs

Lab (initial): $135.
Office (initial): $150.
Supplements: $100.

Method of Payment

Cash and checks are accepted. Insurance is filed. Medicare covers only laboratory fees.

Douglas Brodie, M.D.

848 Tanager
(Mailing Address: P.O. Drawer BL)
Incline Village, Nevada 89450
United States

(702) 832–7001
Fax: (702) 831–5535

Directions

From Reno go south on 395 to Mount Rose Highway (431). Turn right on 431 to state route 28. Turn left and go one mile to Incline Village. At second stop light, turn right; go one short block to Tanager. Turn right onto Tanager. Number 848, or Tanager Square, is on the third block, on the right-hand side.

Background

This clinic provides outpatient care. On the patient's first visit, he or she is initially interviewed by a registered nurse. Then the patient sees a doctor and gets an exam and lab work done. This includes blood, urine, chemistry, darkfield, and homeopathic evaluations. Dr. Brodie has been associated with other well-known physicians in the alternative health care field, such as Dr. John Richardson. Dr Brodie has been using and improving upon these therapies for about 18 years, with a high rate of improvement/remission.

Illness Treated

Cancer; the best responders are pancreas, bladder, prostate, kidney, stomach, some brain tumors, some lung tumors, and breast tumors that have not been operated on or biopsied. The clinic also treats arthritis and arteriosclerosis.

Treatment Offered

Immune system enhancement through vitamins, diet, and amygdalin; amino acid combinations; supplements; and polypeptides derived from thymus, liver, and placenta which activate T-cells and other aspects of the immune system.

Therapy can begin on the first visit with intravenous injections of amygdalin and other supportive supplements to restore immune function and relieve pain. This treatment continues for 21 days with a two-month maintenance program following. Other procedures are employed as well.

Related Readings

Thymus Extrakt Information by Dr. Angel Angelov, West Germany.

Thymic Hormones by Dr. T.D. Luckey, 1973.

The Thymus in Immunity by Dr. J.A.F. Miller. Biol. Basis of Med.

Thymus Factors in Immunity by Dr. H. Friedman. New York Academy of Sciences.

The clinic will also furnish upon request information regarding past patients.

Length of Treatment/Stay

Recommended stay is 21 days. Minimum stay is seven days.

Costs

$4,500 for the 21-day program or $1,500 per week. This does not include food and lodging. Discounts are given at three local motels. The fee does include examinations, lab work, intravenous infusions, peptide injections, and oral or injectable supplements. Maintenance and follow-up are extra.

Method of Payment

Cash, cashier's checks, traveler's checks, and personal checks are accepted. Some insurance companies will pay part of these costs, such as laboratory work, initial examination, and office visits. Medicare does not cover any of these services.

Burzynski Research Institute

Outpatient Clinic:
6221 Corporate Drive
Houston, Texas 77036
United States

(713) 777–8233

Research Institute:
12707 Trinity Drive
Stafford, Texas 77477
United States

(713) 240–5227

Contact Person

Michelle May or Debbie James.

Primary Personnel

Stanislaw R. Burzynski, M.D., Ph.D.

Background

Dr. Burzynski is a physician and biochemist who began his work 24 years ago with a group of peptide growth inhibitors, short chains of amino acids found throughout our bodies which protect us by controlling growth. He discovered a marked deficiency of these peptides in cancer patients.

After leaving Poland in 1970, and while a researcher at Baylor College of Medicine, in part under a grant from the National Cancer Institute, Dr. Burzynski named these peptides "antineoplastons" because of their activity in inhibiting neoplastic, or cancerous, cell growth.

According to the research of Dr. Burzynski and scientists independent of him, his therapy does not work by stimulating the immune system, as many others do. Instead, antineoplastons are components of a biochemical defense system that parallels our immune system. Unlike the immune system, which protects us by destroying invading agents or defective cells, the biochemical defense system protects us by reprogramming, or normalizing, defective cells. Errors in cell programming may lead to such diverse disorders as cancer, benign tumors, certain skin diseases, AIDS, and Parkinson's disease. In 1977, when Dr. Burzynski decided it was time to begin testing on humans, the funds disappeared, so he left Baylor and established his own research facility and outpatient clinic, with privileges at a nearby hospital.

While under treatment, patients undergo careful evaluations, including tumor measurements and appropriate radiologic studies. In addition, a total laboratory profile is taken; it includes a complete blood count, reticulocyte count, urinalysis, determination of carcinoembryonic antigen and other tumor markers, prothrombin time, partial thromboplastin time, indirect and direct Coombs, and a complete blood chemistry profile (SMAC). All patients are treated on an outpatient basis.

The treatment is self-administered and normally free of side effects. For the first two to three weeks of treatment, patients are carefully observed, with appointments scheduled usually at least twice a week, depending on individual progress. Follow-up visits are then scheduled every four to six weeks and average two to five days in length.

Illness Treated

Cancer; the best responders are malignant brain cancers (astrocytoma stages III and IV, and glioblastoma), prostate cancer, lymphoma, and bladder cancer. The clinic is conducting a closed phase II trial for people with AIDS.

Treatment Offered

Patients take antineoplaston treatment either by injection or orally in the form of capsules. Patients who require injections are given antineoplastons several times a day through a catheter in a vein, medically inserted under the clavicle, or by intravenous drip through an intravenous catheter and ambulatory pump. Most of the patients are treated with synthetic antineoplastons, but some are given antineoplastons that have been isolated from healthy human urine. A number of patients since 1977 have accomplished complete remission and cure of cancer.

Related Readings

Antineoplastons (1) Drugs Under Experimental and Clinical Research. Supl. 1, Vol. 12, 1986. Bioscience Ediprint Inc., Geneva, Switzerland.

Antineoplastons (2) Drugs Under Experimental and Clinical Research. Supl. 1, Vol. 13, 1986. Bioscience Ediprint Inc., Geneva, Switzerland.

Length of Treatment/Stay

Initial visit, two to three weeks. Follow-up visits, three- to five-day stays every six to eight weeks.

Costs

Initial consultation: $125.
Apartment rental: contact Monika Szopa at the clinic for current housing costs.
Antineoplaston treatment (includes office visits): from $135 to $685 per day.
Additional costs: housing, transportation, meals, diagnostic tests. Intravenous supplies may also be necessary if that is the determined route of administration for the treatment.

Method of Payment

Cashier's checks, money orders, traveler's checks, and personal checks are accepted. Bring all information regarding insurance policy—group number, identification number, mailing address, and telephone number.

Before starting treatment, the clinic requires an initial $5,000 deposit. After the first week of treatment, the clinic staff will begin filing claims to the patient's insurance company. The ongoing treatment plan will be determined after the first two weeks. That, in turn, will determine the minimum deposits, which can range from $3,000 to $5,000 per month until insurance begins payments.

Once insurance begins making substantial payments, the patient will no longer be required to make monthly deposits. The initial deposit will be refunded at the end of treatment when insurance has paid 100% of the bill. If insurance payments are interrupted during treatment, the patient will be responsible for the monthly deposits until insurance payments resume.

Harold E. Buttram, M.D.

5724 Clymer Road
Quakertown, Pennsylvania 18951
United States

(215) 536–1891
(215) 536–1700

Primary Personnel

Harold E. Buttram, M.D.

Background

Dr. Buttram is an internist who practices holistic medical care, comprising nutritional, metabolic, and immunotherapy.

Illness Treated

Cancer or other chronic degenerative and auto-immune disorders.

Treatment Offered

Botanicals, anti-oxidents, enzymes, detoxification, lab testing of immune and tumor activity, chelation, clinical ecology, intravenous support, and dietetics.

Length of Treatment/Stay

Depends upon specific illness, effects of prior treatment, and state of immune system.

Costs

Initial extended consultation costs $150. Other costs, though not submitted for publication, depend upon the severity of the illness and on prior and current treatments.

Cancer Treatment Centers of America

(800) FOR HELP (24 hours)

Affiliated Hospitals:

American International Hospital
Shiloh Boulevard & Emmaus Avenue
Zion, Illinois 60099
United States

(708) 872–4561

Memorial Medical Center and Cancer Institute
8181 South Lewis Avenue
Tulsa, Oklahoma 74137
United States

(918) 496–5000

Background

Cancer Treatment Centers of America is a network of facilities dedicated to the treatment of one disease—cancer. Two hospital-based centers are in operation, one in Zion, Illinois, about 40 miles north of Chicago, and the other in Tulsa, Oklahoma. The centers draw patients from across the country and around the world with a mix of traditional and alternative treatments and services.

Illness Treated

Cancer.

Treatment Offered

Alternative therapies, including whole body and localized hyperthermia, as well as fractionated dose chemotherapy, which minimizes or eliminates many side effects. In addition, the centers stress nutrition, the "mind-body connection," and the spiritual aspects of healing and health. Along with these treatment modalities, the overall team approach makes the patients the focus of the decision-making process, maximizing their ability and right to make informed choices.

Length of Treatment/Stay

Depends upon patient, but treatment is based on inpatient visits.

Costs

Costs not submitted for publication.

Center for Metabolic Disorders

5030 90th Way S.W.
Fort Lauderdale, Florida 33328
United States

CA Laboratory:
1818 Sheridan Street
Hollywood, Florida 33020
United States

(305) 929–4814

Primary Personnel

E.K. Schandl, Ph.D., F.A.C.B.

Directions

One mile west of Hollywood Beach on the Atlantic coast.

Background

The CA Laboratory has developed a biochemical cancer profile done on a small vial of blood which they claim can monitor the progress of cancer therapy and possibly foretell the development of malignancies more than two years prior to diagnosis.

In conjunction with Human Hospital in Hollywood, Florida, they offer an acute care facility. They use metabolic therapy as the main modality and surgery when needed, after preparation with vitamin C.

Dr. Schandl also offers biochemical/nutritional consultations, which can be used to create metabolic programs for rehabilitation and improvement.

Illness Treated

Cancer, heart disease, multiple sclerosis, Parkinson's disease, viral and bacterial infections, lupus, malabsorption syndromes, AIDS, chronic fatigue, and candidiasis.

Treatment Offered

Metabolic-IV vitamin C, interferon, hyperbaric oxygen, colon therapy, physical therapy, nutritional therapy, and orthodox medical treatments, if necessary. For the CA Laboratory profile, contact the laboratory for instructions on what to send and how to send it.

Length of Treatment/Stay

Tests are reported weekly; hospital stay averages two weeks.

Costs

Blood workup: $139 to $224.
Consultation: $95.
Hospital fees, IV therapy, and other therapies would all cost extra.

Method of Payment

For blood tests, only money orders are accepted. At the hospital, other methods of payment are accepted. Insurance may cover 80% of fees.

Center for Preventive Medicine and Dentistry

111 Bala Avenue
Bala Cynwyd, Pennsylvania 19004
United States

(215) 667–2927

Primary Personnel

Howard Posner, M.D., medical director.

Directions

From Route 76 (Schulkill Expressway), take City Avenue exit (also Route 1 south). After about one mile, turn right on Bala Avenue (a Mellon Bank is on the corner). Coming from Route 1 south, Bala Avenue is about two miles on the left after crossing Route 30 (Lancaster Avenue). The center is on the second block on the right side of the street.

Background

This center has on its staff a doctor, nutritionist, dentist, chiropractor, and ophthalmologist all working together in a healing environment, using preventive approaches to health.

Illness Treated

Cancer, degenerative diseases, chronic fatigue, yeast infection, depression, arthritis, heart disease, and hypertension.

Treatment Offered

Some types of treatment given are nutritional supplements, herbs, visualization, stress management, and, if necessary, prescription drugs.

Costs

$40 for a full visit.

Method of Payment

Cash, checks, Visa, MasterCard, and American Express are accepted. For medical treatment, most insurance companies cover costs. Payment is requested at time of visit, and the insurance company will reimburse.

Centro Medico Arturo Toledo

Immunotherapy Unit
Paseo Playas de Tijuana 105
Playas de Tijuana, B.C. 22700
Mexico

Mailing Address:
P.O. Box 430713
San Diego, California 92143–0713
United States

(690) 690–1576
(800) 541–8160

Contact Person

Silvia, Laura, or Lucy.

Primary Personnel

Jose L. Lepe-Zuniga, M.D., Ph.D. (doctor in immunology).

Directions

From San Diego, take I-5 south to Tijuana. Once crossing the border follow the signs to Rosarito-Ensenada, exit in Playas (6 miles), and go straight. The clinic is on the left-hand side on Paseo Playas about a third of a mile after yellow flashing lights.

Background

The fundamental concept is that the immune system of every person is intrinsically capable of recognizing malignant cells and destroying them in a selective fashion. The manipulation or modification of the immune balance to achieve this goal is called immunotherapy. Dr. Lepe-Zuniga has been researching immunological ways to treat cancer and other diseases for more than ten years, developing a sense of what to do and what not to do to a cancer patient. He is essentially opposed to chemotherapy for the treatment of most forms of advanced cancer and recognizes the importance of nutrition and personal attitude in the healing process.

Illness Treated

Cancer (with or without metastasis); best responders are carcinomas (kidney, breast, colon, prostate, stomach, pancreas, ovary, and others), followed by melanomas and sarcomas. Leukemias and lymphomas are treated by a combination of conventional treatment and immunotherapy. The unit has also developed treatments for chronic fatigue syndrome, psoriasis, chronic hepatitis B, chronic yeast infections, and autoimmune disorders such as systemic lupus, rheumatoid arthritis, multiple sclerosis, aplastic anemia, and purpuras. Brain tumors and primary lung cancer (advanced) are not treated.

Treatment Offered

A three-phase therapeutic approach to cancer. First, patients undergo plasmapheresis (plasma exchange) to remove from the blood any tumor-derived substances. In the second phase, the immune response against the tumor is induced by activating the immune cells with natural substances in the presence of tumoral cells. In the third phase, the initial immune response is amplified to levels at which the tumor is rejected from the body. The treatment is supplemented by a special diet, vitamins, and enzymes. The center claims that patients who respond will be cured completely from the particular cancer they suffer. Information on treatment for other diseases is provided upon request.

Related Readings

"Cellular Immunity Against Tumor Antigens" by K.E. Hellstrom and I. Hellstrom. In *Advanced Cancer Research*, 1969.

"The Concept of Immunological Surveillance" by F.M. Burnet. In *Prog. Experimental Tumor Research*, 1970.

"Cellular and Cytokine Immunotherapy of Cancer" by J.M. Cruse and R.E. Lewis Jr. In *Prog. Experimental Tumor Research*, 1988.

"Plasma Exchange in Cancer Patients" by L. Israel, R. Edelstein, R. Samak, et al. In *Immunotherapy of Malignant Diseases* by H. Rainer (editor). F.K. Schattauer Verlag. Stuttgart. 1978.

Length of Treatment/Stay

The whole treatment is given in a small general hospital during a period of seven to ten days. Follow-up is monthly for three months, during which complete cure should take place.

Costs

Initial evaluation for eligibility: $50 (laboratory and X-ray fees not included). Complete treatment: $7,000, which includes a ten-day hospital stay, two plasma exchanges, all biologicals, medicines (including albumin and IV solutions) for the treatment itself, laboratory testing before and during treatment, electrocardiogram, two chest X-rays, and all medical fees (except for surgeons or other specialists who might be called upon).

Method of Payment

Cash (in United States dollars), traveler's checks, certified checks, and money orders. Coverage by insurance is investigated. Payment in full is requested in advance.

Cose Inc.

(Centre d'Orthobiologie Somatidienne de l'Estrie Inc.)

5270 Rue Fontaine
Rock Forest, Quebec, J1N 3B6
Canada

(819) 564–7883
Fax: (819) 564–4668
Fax: (819) 564–2195

Primary Personnel

Gaston Naessens, Françoise Naessens, Stéphane Sdicu, Daniel Sdicu, André Sdicu.

Background

More than 40 years ago, Gaston Naessens invented the Somatoscope, a darkfield microscope capable of reaching 30,000× magnification with a 150-angstrom resolution on living particles. The Somatoscope makes it possible to observe processes in freshly extracted blood and to view its subcellular particles. Gaston Naessens hypothesizes that all living beings, animal and vegetable, possess life by virtue of tiny specks of crystalized life which he calls "somatids." His unique approach to diagnosing cancer patients relies a good deal on using his Somatoscope to view the somatids in the blood. (Orthodox medicine has no blood test for cancer.) He believes cancer stems from nitrogen starvation in the body.

Illness Treated

Cancer, chronic fatigue syndrome, arthritis, and all other degenerative diseases.

Treatment Offered

714X (trimethylbicyclonitraminoheptane chloride). This medicine is a camphor-derivate nitrogen with mineral salts. The goal is to restore nitrogen to the tissues that have been deprived of it. The medicine has no side effects. It should be used only with the supervision of a physician.

Related Readings

The Persecution and Trial of Gaston Naessens by Christopher Bird, 1991.

The Galileo of the Microscope by Christopher Bird, 1990.

AIDS, Cancer, and the Medical Establishment by Dr. Raymond Keith Brown, 1986.

Somatids: The Theory and Technique, Part I. This is a 55-minute VHS videocassette of broadcast quality.

Length of Treatment

714X is injected daily (perinodular). A series of shots consists of 21 daily injections; three such series are the minimum required, but most patients should expect to undergo longer-term treatment.

Costs

$320 in United States funds for enough medicine for one series of shots. Delivery takes only a few days. Included with the medicine are a protocol, injection instructions, and a videocassette on the treatment.

Method of Payment

Payment must be accompanied by a medical prescription. Checks and money orders made out to Cose Inc. are accepted. The medicine will not be mailed to post office boxes. Full name, address, and telephone number must accompany prescription and payment.

Falk Oncology Centre Ltd.

111 Wellesley Street East (3rd Floor)
Toronto, Ontario M4Y 2Y2
Canada

(416) 593–4713

Contact Person

Rudolf E. Falk, M.D.

Primary Personnel

Rudolf E. Falk, M.D.

Directions

Located in downtown Toronto at the corner of Wellesley and Jarvis Streets.

Background

The centre, established by Dr. Rudy Falk in September 1985, is dedicated to the development of innovative therapies for the increasing number of cancer patients, many of whom are unresponsive to standard cancer treatment. Dr. Falk founded the Goldie Rotman Cancer Clinic in 1978 and remains director of surgical oncology at Toronto General Hospital. He is also experienced in neurosurgery and transplantation. He is a professor of surgery and pathology at the University of Toronto and has been a career investigator for the Medical Research Council of Canada since 1973.

The centre operates on an outpatient basis. It treats up to 60 patients a day and sees as many as 20 new patients a week.

Illness Treated

Cancer; the best responses are being seen in all solid tumors (regardless of previous treatment), including non-small cell carcinoma of the lung, hepatoma, and sarcoma.

Treatment Offered

NSAID drugs with a carrier/penetrating agent to decrease side effects. This is a safe procedure. The drugs have been shown to block excessive production of prostaglandin, which appears to be present in all experimental and clinical tumors. The drugs improve the patient's own immune reaction to the tumor. Treatment at the centre is expected to begin a response;

the patient then follows up the treatment at home with intermittent intravenous infusions of NSAIDs with the carrier/penetrating molecule. Less and less cytotoxic therapy and hyperthermia is being used.

Related Readings

Contact centre for extensive list of Dr. Falk's publications.

Length of Treatment/Stay

Five to seven days approximately once per month.

Costs

$500–$1,500 (Canadian) per day of treatment. Actual amount depends on the type of tumor, previous treatment, and extensiveness of the disease.

Method of Payment

Checks, cash, Visa, and money orders are accepted. Major insurance companies cover costs.

Yolanda Fraire, M.D.

Calle 8 #1941–A
(Entre Revolucion and Madero)
4th Floor
Tijuana, B.C.
Mexico

0 (115) 266–89–2104

Primary Personnel

Yolanda Fraire, M.D.

Directions

After crossing the border, follow 3rd Avenue. Take the downtown exit to Revolution Avenue and turn left to 8th Street. Office is located between Revolution Avenue and Madero, next to the Sanborn's store, which offers underground parking. Her office is on the fourth floor.

Background

Dr. Fraire was chief doctor at the Hoxsey Clinic for many years. She graduated from medical school at the Autonomous University of Coahuila in 1971 and worked at the Bio-Medical Center from 1973 to 1985. Her office is an outpatient facility.

Illness Treated

Cancer, chronic degenerative diseases, immunity suppression, Candida albicans. Best cancer results are with metastatic breast cancer, metastatic prostate cancer, lymphoma, colon cancer, and lung cancer.

Treatment Offered

Allopathic and homeopathic medicines, including Formula 86, anti-fungal vaccine, nystain, diet, staphage-lysate, isoprinosine, cimetidine, indomethacine, and butyrate.

Treatment starts with a clinical history and a thorough examination. An initial evaluation is made of the patient's health. Subdermal skin tests with Candida antigen and staphage-lysate are then administered, and complete laboratory testing is done (cancer test, immune tests, blood chemistry, blood-cell count, serotypology, stool studies, urine analysis, and, if necessary, X-rays). A complete evaluation of the patient's health is then made, and a modality of treatment is chosen. The patient is released with a six-month supply of medication. Periodic check-ups are advised.

Length of Treatment/Stay

Evaluation and examination takes three to four days, two or three hours per day. Appointments are necessary. Patients should bring 90-minute cassettes for recording each daily session.

Costs

Approximately $4,000 for six months of treatment, including the physical, some lab and X-ray studies, and the medicine. Room, board, and transportation are not provided, but the doctor will advise you of the most convenient arrangements.

Method of Payment

Money orders, traveler's checks, and cashier's checks are preferred. Credit cards are not accepted.

GAM Diagnostic Nutritional Medical Center

975 Ryland Street
Reno, Nevada 89502
United States

(800) 732–0837
(702) 324–6900

Primary Personnel

Vera J. Allison, N.M.D., founder; James W. Forsythe, M.D., consulting and referral.

Directions

The medical center is minutes away from Reno International Airport.

Background

Dr. Allison graduated from the Pacific College of Naturopathic Medicine in southern California in 1958 and was one of the first naturopaths to be licensed in the state of Nevada. Dr. Forsythe is surgeon general of Nevada, as well as a hemotologist, pathologist, oncologist, and doctor of internal medicine.

Dr. Allison is a protégée of the late Dr. Ernst T. Krebs Sr., a pioneer in the use of laetrile in the treatment of cancer. She later worked with his son, Dr. Byron Krebs, who also treated patients with laetrile. Dr. Allison's work in this field spans 30 years.

Illness Treated

Cancer; specializes in inoperable brain tumors, diabetes, arthritis, multiple sclerosis, and other degenerative diseases.

Treatment Offered

Metabolic, nutritional, noninvasive stone dissolution, balancing of body chemistry, colon therapy, acu-therapy, reflexology, advanced antiviral therapy, craniology, computer augmented diagnosis, massage, and individualized metabolic programs for the management of degenerative disease. The center also offers the Heitan–La Garde–Bradford blood test, which uses a specially designed phase-contrast microscope to view changes in coagulated blood structure associated with degenerative diseases.

Length of Treatment/Stay

Three to four weeks, average. Sometimes six weeks, for brain or bone cancer.

Costs

Varies; the average is $4,000–$6,000. Brain or bone cancer: $8,000–$10,000.

Method of Payment

Cash, cashier's checks, Visa, MasterCard, and American Express are accepted. Some insurance will pay for a percentage of the treatment, but check with the center first.

Gerson Therapy— Hospital De Baja, California

Gerson Institute:
P.O. Box 430
Bonita, California 91908
United States

(619) 472–7450

Centro Hospitalario del Pacifico S.A. (CHIPSA):
No. 449 Nubes
Playas de Tijuana, B.C.
Mexico

Contact Person

Charlotte Gerson; Gar Hildenbrand; Norman Fritz.

Primary Personnel

Seven medical doctors, nursing staff, etc.

Directions

After crossing the United States border into Mexico, take the Ensenada toll road and exit on the Playas off ramp.

Background

Charlotte Gerson teaches the therapy that her father, Max Gerson, M.D, founded in Germany and New York. The hospital is located in Tijuana near the beach. Reservations are suggested for this inpatient facility. Patients and their companions may stay in one of many rooms with a private bath. Gerson therapy has been in Mexico for 14 years. It has just moved into a modern, multilevel, 48-bed hospital (CHIPSA). Although this therapy requires a great deal of work to maintain, it is said to be good for "incurable degenerative diseases where the patient's body has not been poisoned by other treatments." For absolute recovery, compliance with the Gerson diet is recommended for one and a half years. Because the Gerson therapy is most difficult to undertake, it is considered unwise to begin the treatment unless one is able to follow through for the one and a half to two years necessary. Evaluations were published three times in 1990, in *Contemporary Nutritional Medicine* (Germany), Lechner, April 1990; in *The Lancet* (Great Britain), James, September 1990; and in "Unconventional Cancer Treatments," U.S. Congress-OTA, September 1990.

Illness Treated

All types of cancer respond. Metastasized melanoma, lung cancers, bladder and kidney cancers, lymphoma, and pancreas and liver cancers respond exceptionally well; improvements are frequently rapid and dramatic. The center also treats multiple sclerosis, diabetes, arthritis and other degenerative diseases, drug addiction, and (in a preventive, not a curative approach) AIDS.

Treatment Offered

Intensive detoxification and nutrition program. The Gerson therapy involves: 13 raw, freshly pressed juices daily, at hourly intervals, consisting of organic carrots and apples, and green vegetables; three meals a day of organically grown foods low in protein, salt, and fat (cooked vegetables, raw salads, fresh fruits); coffee enemas; dietary supplements of potassium iodide, enzymes, thyroid, Lugol (iodine), niacin, and crude liver extract; and vitamin B_{12} injections.

This therapy emphasizes the potassium-sodium balance within the cells and fluids of the body. The institute also uses ozone therapy, intravenous potassium, laetrile, Koch, clay, etc., adjunctively.

Related Readings

Cancer: A Healing Crisis by Jack Tropp. Exposition Press, 1980.

A Cancer Therapy: Results of 50 Cases by Max Gerson, M.D. Gerson Institute, 1986.

Cancer Winner by Jacquie Davison. Gerson Institute, 1989.

Censured for Curing Cancer by S.J. Haught. Gerson Institute, 1983.

Healing Journal. Gerson Institute.

A Time To Heal by Beata Bishop. 1985. (U.S. title: *My Triumph Over Cancer.*)

A mail-order catalog of books and cassette tapes is available upon request. A list of survivors with photos is given in the brochure.

Length of Treatment/Stay

A minimum stay is two weeks. A stay of three to eight weeks is recommended.

Costs

Weekly deposit: $3,990 ($495 per day plus 15% tax). Lab tests: $200 and up per week, depending on the individual. Recommended to have companion to help; cost is $322 per week ($40 per day plus 15% tax).

Method of Payment

Payment must be in cash or traveler's checks only. Many private insurance companies will reimburse the patient. Hospital management requires prepayment.

Gibson Clinic of Preventive Medicine

215 North Third Street
Ponca City, Oklahoma 74601
United States

(405) 762–5746

Primary Personnel

Robert W. Gibson, M.D.

Directions

From I-35, take Tonkowa exit 17 and go 13 miles straight east on four-lane highway to Ponca City.

Background

The clinic was established in 1920 by Dr. Gibson (Sr.) and is now run by his son, who has been specializing in preventive medicine since the early 1950s.

Illness Treated

Cancer and other diseases.

Treatment Offered

Nutrition, vitamins, enzymes, and laetrile. The center has been using its methods for more than 11 years.

Length of Treatment/Stay

Eighteen days. The center is an outpatient clinic.

Costs

$3,000 for three weeks.

Method of Payment

Cash and checks are accepted. Although the center does not accept insurance, it will help the patient file for reimbursement.

David P. Goldberg, D.O., and Associates Inc.

100 Forest Park Drive
Dayton, Ohio 45404
United States

(513) 277–1722
(513) 274–1169

Offices:
2468 Dayton-Xenia Road
Beavercreek, Ohio 45385
United States

(513) 426–4276

116 Commerce Street
Lewisberg, Ohio 48338
United States

(513) 962–2488

Contact Person

Gerda, head nurse.

Primary Personnel

David Goldberg, D.O.; Robert Gardner, D.O.; Paul Martin, D.O.; Carl Hoyng, D.O.

Directions

I-75 to Needmore exit, go west on Needmore, turn left onto Riverside Drive. Right at first traffic light. You will enter the back of a parking lot. Go left and you will see a one-story brick building with a brown roof. That is the office.

Background

Office offers a general practice, laser surgery, osteopathic manipulation, preventive medicine, chelation therapy, counseling, and other holistic procedures.

Illness Treated

Cancer and others.

Treatment Offered

B_{17}, intravenous treatments, nutritional treatments.

Costs

Intravenous treatment: $75 to $95, depending on formula.
B_{17} must be obtained by the patient.

Nutritional treatment: $28 for office visit, vitamins, and supplements.
Payment is due when the services are rendered.

Method of Payment

MasterCard, Visa, personal checks, and cash are accepted.

Nicholas Gonzalez, M.D.

737 Park Avenue
New York, New York 10021
United States

(212) 535–3993

Primary Personnel

Nicholas Gonzalez, M.D.

Directions

The clinic is located in mid-Manhattan.

Background

Dr. Gonzalez has a B.A. from Brown University. He has done postgraduate work at Columbia University and received an M.D. from Cornell University. He has specialty training in clinical immunology. His fellowship was completed under Dr. Robert A. Good.

Dr. Gonzalez has a private practice, working in association with a small group of well-trained physicians. His own specialty training is in clinical immunology, although his current interest relates to nutrition. He has no inpatient facilities.

Illness Treated

Cancer, most degenerative diseases, and AIDS.

Treatment Offered

An intensive nutritional approach based on the methods of Dr. William Kelley. Dr. Gonzalez performed a six-year investigation of Dr. Kelley's success in over 10,000 patients.

Related Readings

The results of Dr. Gonzalez's study are in book form and are available to interested professional people as well as patients.

Length of Treatment/Stay

A two-day evaluation in New York is required. Patients follow the program at home.

Costs

Approximately $4,000–$5,000 for a year of treatment, including the cost of supplements.

Method of Payment

Cash, checks, money orders, Blue Cross, Blue Shield, and other types of insurance are accepted.

Health Restoration Center

22821 Lake Forest Drive, Suite 114
El Toro, California 92630
United States

(714) 770–9616

Contact Person

Noyemy.

Primary Personnel

David Steenblock, D.O.

Directions

Interstate 5 between San Diego and Los Angeles. Turn east on Lake Forest Drive, go one and a half blocks to Aspen, turn left, then turn right into first parking lot in the Aspen Plaza.

Background

This general outpatient medical clinic is about 11 years old. The clinic's primary focus is on using non-painful therapy to restore a person's health. If patients are undergoing chemotherapy or radiation therapy, the doctor will work closely with them to reduce and/or eliminate the toxic side effects and to rebuild their weakened bodies and immune systems.

Illness Treated

Cancer and other diseases.

Treatment Offered

Nutrition, chelation, cryosurgery (freezing tumors), herbology, homeopathy, isopathy, vitamin therapy, hormonal therapy, immunological therapy, hyperbaric oxygen, urea, and allergy work.

Related Readings

Dr. Steenblock has written many articles in *Let's Live* and *Total Health*. Dr. Steenblock has also published *Chlorella, Natural Medicinal Algae*, a review of the world's scientific research on the healing effects of chlorella. For a list of all articles, videotapes, and books available, send a self-addressed envelope to the center.

Length of Treatment/Stay

One month, with follow-ups.

Costs

Initial costs are $500–$1,000, most of which is covered by insurance. The treatment then costs $300–$2,000 per month, depending on the nature, extent, and severity of the disease. Most of the monthly cost is not covered by insurance.

Method of Payment

Cash, personal checks, traveler's checks, Visa, and MasterCard are accepted. Most therapies are recognized by insurance companies.

Holistic Medical Center

8760 Sunset Boulevard
Los Angeles, California 90069
United States

(213) 854–0404

Contact Person

Emil Levin, M.D.

Primary Personnel

Emil Levin, M.D.

Directions

From West Hollywood, take La Cienega heading north, turn left onto Sunset Boulevard, heading west. The center is a little before Holloway Drive.

Background

The clinic has 10,000 square feet of ecologically balanced office space. Dr. Levin is a graduate of USSR Medical School with training in internal medicine. He spent three years in New York and has been at his present location for three years. His is a holistic-eclectic practice utilizing the newest developments of German diagnostic and therapeutic homeopathic techniques. Emphasis is on the biochemical balancing of vitamins and minerals. Dr. Levin is a vice president in the International League of Doctors Against Vivisection.

Illness Treated

Cancer and other degenerative diseases (diabetes, vascular disorders, arthritis, etc.) as well as AIDS. Holistic parasitology, viral illnesses, and food and environmental allergies. Also, learning problems, pediatric nutrition problems, and brain dysfunction.

Treatment Offered

Colon hydrotherapy, chelation therapy, allergy desensitization-homeopathic phenolic dilutions, vitamin-mineral balancing. Patients are accepted only after handwritten doctor/patient agreement is filled out. Side effects of the treatment are extremely rare and are quickly and completely reversible. Dietary demands are very strict.

Related Readings

Journal of Orthomolecular Medicine.

Psychiatry.

All works of John Bastyr College of Naturopathy.

Energy by Dr. Paul Eck.

Townsend Letter for Doctors.

Length of Treatment/Stay

For best results, biweekly visits to the clinic for treatments (not doctor's visits) are recommended.

Costs

Varies from case to case, but physical exam, first visit, blood tests, tissue mineral analysis test, and homeopathic diagnostic screening are all required. For many degenerative diseases, a realistic price would be $5,000 to $7,000.

Method of Payment

Cash and money orders are accepted. All insurance forms are promptly filled out.

Hospital Ernesto Contreras

Paseo de Tijuana #1
Playas de Tijuana, B.C. 22700
Mexico

011–526–680–1850
　　800–326–1850
　　619–428–6438
　　619–428–4486
Fax: 011–526–680–2709

Mailing Address:
P.O. Box 439045
San Diego, California 92143–9045
United States

Contact Person

For medical information, write or call Dr. Contreras. For appointments, estimates, insurance questions, and other information, call the public relations office.

Primary Personnel

Dr. Ernesto Contreras Sr., general director and founder; Dr. Ernesto Contreras Jr., medical director and oncologist; Dr. Francisco Contreras, general administrator and surgeon.

Directions

If you are driving, after crossing the border take the lane with the sign "Rosarita Ensenada." Follow it without changing lanes. After several turns it will lead you to Rosarita Ensenada Toll Highway. Drive west about six miles. When you get close to the ocean, take the right lane, which goes to the beach (playas). Half a mile farther, you will see the big bull ring. Across the street from it is Hospital Ernesto Contreras.

If you are flying, book your flight to San Diego International Airport. Call the hospital's receptionist ahead of time and tell her the airline, flight number, and day and time of arrival. A driver from the hospital will meet you at the luggage claim area.

Background

Dr. Ernesto Contreras Sr. has completed 50 years of medical practice. He has devoted his past 30 years to finding less-aggressive but more-effective alternatives for the treatment of cancer. He is assisted by his two sons, who are medical doctors and cancer specialists, and by health care professionals. Facilities include a 50-bed hospital, outpatient accommodations, a pharmacy, a clinical laboratory, a radiology department, and a cafeteria that serves a special diet to the patients. Hospital Ernesto Contreras is the largest comprehensive cancer center in northwestern Mexico.

Illness Treated

Cancer; also, most chronic degenerative diseases, such as arthritis, multiple sclerosis, and lupus.

Treatment Offered

Metabolic therapy, using amygdalin (laetrile), enzymes, and megadoses of vitamins A and C; Alivett therapy, using the original Greek formula from the late Dr. Hariton Alivizatos; Warburg therapy, using a formula developed by Dr. Cone; 714X therapy, using a vaccine developed by Dr. Gaston Naessens of Canada; live cell therapy; shark cartilage; Immusyn-C; vitamin and mineral megadoses; etc. All the programs are nontoxic and use a special diet, detoxification, and immuno-modulators.

Part of the therapy involves the use of psychological and spiritual methods to build up the immune system. In the nearby San Pueblo Christian Community Church, religious services in English are offered to patients and relatives on Sundays from 10 a.m. to noon. Dr. Contreras Sr. also conducts bible studies.

Also offered is a cancer prevention program that includes the Arthur (AMID) test.

Related Readings

Amygdalin, a monographic study. Kem S.A. Laboratories.

Length of Treatment/Stay

The average is three to four weeks.

Costs

For the metabolic and the Warburg programs, the average cost is $6,500 to $10,000, including room and board. The average cost for the Alivett program is $2,400, but those patients will also have to pay for their motel room and meals. Patients can keep their costs down by bringing copies of their medical records and X-rays.

Method of Payment

Cash, traveler's checks, and money orders are accepted. Credit cards and personal checks are not accepted. Private insurance companies accept claims in most cases.

Hospital Santa Monica

Rosarito Beach B.C.
Mexico

Mailing Address:
424 Calle Primera
Suite 102
San Ysidro, California 92173
United States

(619) 428–1147 (answered by Wellness Lifestyle)

Primary Personnel

Kurt W. Donsbach, Ph.D.; Humberto Seimunde, M.D., chief of staff.

Directions

Just north of Rosarito Beach. Call for specific directions.

Background

This modern two-story hospital on the Pacific has sixty beds; forty-six have ocean views. This program has been available for more than seven years and is part of an international group, with sister hospitals in Poland and Russia. Hospital Santa Monica has integrated therapies for cancer and other diseases from all over the world and offers what it considers the most comprehensive programs available. Its founder, Dr. Kurt Donsbach, has pioneered several therapies, including intravenous hydrogen peroxide. A full laboratory and emergency facilities are on the premises.

Illness Treated

Cancer, arthritis, allergies, multiple sclerosis, candidiasis, cardiovascular disease, and chronic degenerative disease.

Treatment Offered

Intravenous infusions that include free amino acids to help rebuild the cells; vitamins and minerals to act as a sparkplug to get things going; GH3 as a cellular rejuvenant; DMSO to help transport other materials into the cell; hydrogen peroxide to destroy candida and other unwanted intruders; live cell therapy; laetrile and eleven other substances; EDTA where indicated to relieve cardiovascular disorders; and super oxide dismutase for special conditions. Colonics, ozone, and other immune stimulating medicines are also available. The hospital has a dentist for amalgam removal on the premises and an extensive physical therapy department in which pulsed biomagnetic therapy is offered. Counseling is always available.

Related Readings

The clinic will furnish upon request information regarding past patients (but not patient telephone numbers, because of privacy reasons). Several videocassettes of cured patients are available.

Length of Treatment/Stay

Twenty-one days, with extended care available.

Costs

The total care program for twenty-one days varies from $6,500 to $8,500. This includes a physical exam, all tests, room, meals, cell therapy, all medications, all supplements, additional consultation, and a maintenance program.

Method of Payment

Cashier's checks, money orders, cash, Visa, and MasterCard are accepted. Most private insurance companies will cover at least a considerable portion of the expenses. Medicare does not cover any of the costs.

Richard P. Huemer, M.D.

Cascade Park Health Group Inc.
406 Southeast 131st Avenue
Suite C-303
Vancouver, Washington 98684
United States

(800) 444–1696
(205) 253–4445
(503) 256–9666

Primary Personnel

Richard P. Huemer, M.D.; Paula R. Bickle, Ph.D.

Directions

From Portland International Airport, go north on highway I-205 to Mill Plain, then head east on Mill Plain to 131st Street and turn right.

Background

Dr. Huemer has been involved full-time with nutritional and metabolic therapies since 1974. Previously, he was involved for nine years in research on cancer immunology. The clinic is an outpatient facility.

Illness Treated

Cancer, most degenerative diseases, chemical sensitivities, chronic fatigue, and immune deficiency syndrome.

Treatment Offered

Dr. Huemer does not treat cancer per se, but he provides nutritional support programs for cancer patients under the care of an oncologist. The support includes intravenous vitamin C, high-dose nutrient therapy, and immune stimulation. BCG is used as an adjunctive therapy in selected cases. Possible side effects are local scarring due to the BCG, and toxicity from vitamin A and selenium.

Contact the office for specific instructions on how to prepare for an appointment and the tests that will be part of your first visit.

Related Readings

I Beat Cancer by Bernice Wallin. Contemporary Books, 1978.

Roots of Molecular Medicine by R.P. Huemer (editor). W.H. Freeman, 1986.

"The Healthy Heart Chart" by R.P. Huemer, M. McCarty, and H. Boynton. Nutrition 21, 1985.

Length of Treatment/Stay

Depends upon the situation.

Costs

Charges are based upon the amount of time spent. The initial visit costs about $150, excluding office tests. Lab tests are extra and will be billed directly to you by the lab. Follow-up visits cost about $80. IVs range in price from $75 to $100.

Method of Payment

MasterCard, Visa, and cash are accepted. Cascade Park Health Group will bill insurance carriers. Patients are responsible for charges not covered by insurance. Payment at the time of service is requested for the first visit.

Immune Therapy Clinic

Paseo Ensenada #9
Playas de Tijuana
Tijuana, B.C. 22200
Mexico

011–526–680–6830
Fax: 011–526–680–6861

Mailing Address:
Immune Therapy Clinic
416 West San Ysidro Boulevard
Suite L-702
San Ysidro, California 92073
United States

(619) 428–2211 (24-hour answering service)

Contact Person

Brady Fleck or Olga Leal.

Primary Personnel

Dr. Gustavo Anderade; Brady Fleck.

Directions

The clinic is a 15-minute drive south of San Diego. Take highway I-5 south to the Mexican border. After crossing the border, follow the signs to "Rosarito/Ensenada" for approximately 10 miles. The last exit before the first tollgate on the road to "Rosarito/Ensenada" will be to Playas de Tijuana. Take exit down the hill. Make the first left, around the Denny's restaurant. Go to the end of the block. Go straight through the traffic signal. The clinic is the third building on the left-hand side of the road.

Background

The clinic was established by cancer patients. It tries to stay on the leading edge in the battle against cancer by doing research around the world and by staying outside the United States. It offers treatments from around the world and arranges for the patient's travel to the clinic, accommodations while at the clinic, and, if necessary, a follow-up program for after the patient goes home.

Illness Treated

Cancer, all types, including prostate, breast, brain, lung, colon, lymphoma, and mesothelioma. Specializes in metastatic cancers. Also treats osteoporosis and offers preventive treatment.

Treatment Offered

Immune system stimulation; metabolic; nutritional; and diphosphonate.

Length of Treatment/Stay

Three to eight weeks, depending on the patient's condition and the treatment given. Patients may stay in San Diego or Mexico.

Costs

Evaluation: Free.
Immune stimulation: $5,200 for the first four weeks.
Metabolic treatment: Varies.
Nutritional treatment: Varies.
Diphosphonate: $100 per infusion.
Lodgings: Rates vary, but patients will need to pay the hotel, motel, or campground in which they choose to stay.

Method of Payment

Cash, cashier's checks, and bank wire transfers are accepted. The clinic suggests that patients open a checking account in San Diego.

Immuno-Augmentative Therapy Centre

P.O. Box F-2689
Freeport, Grand Bahama Island
Bahamas

(809) 352–7455/6

IAT Patients' Association Inc.:
Box 10
Otho, Iowa 50569–0010
United States

(515) 972–4444

Primary Personnel

Lawrence Burton, Ph.D.

Directions

Take taxi from airport (approximate cost is $3).

Background

Dr. Burton's outpatient clinic, located in Freeport, Grand Bahama Island, was founded in 1977 as a not-for-profit foundation. He has a well-equipped laboratory and clinic dedicated to providing immuno-augmentative therapy. In addition to bringing a passport or birth certificate, patients must bring a companion. They must stay a minimum of ten to twelve weeks on their first visit.

Rental cars are available, as are taxis and limited bus service. Supermarkets and shops are also accessible. A list is provided upon request of apartments with kitchens to rent during your stay.

Immuno-augmentative therapy is also available in Germany, twenty minutes from Dusseldorf, at the GIT Clinic, A.H. Strassee 22, Gelsenkirken, Germany 4650. The telephone is (49) (209) 208020. The therapy will be available in other countries as well. Check with the Bahamas or the Patients' Association for the latest developments.

The Office of Technology Assessment, a branch of Congress, is evaluating Dr. Burton's treatment.

Illness Treated

Cancer; the best responders are malignant lymphoma, mesothelioma, metastatic colon cancer, brain tumors, squamous cell carcinoma, Hodgkin's disease (often the type not responsive to chemotherapy), and cancer of the cervix, lung, and larynx.

Treatment Offered

Immuno-augmentative therapy. Burton discovered substances in the blood that help the body fight cancer cells. He discovered ways to extract these substances from blood, refine and process them, and reintroduce them into the body.

Related Readings

Cancer Survivors and How They Did It by Judith Glassman. Dial Press, 1983.

The Cancer Syndrome by Ralph Moss (Chapter 12). Grove Press, 1980.

Transcript of the Molinari Hearings available from Congressman Guy Molinari, Fort Wadsworth Building #203, Staten Island, New York 10305.

The centre will also furnish upon request information regarding past patients.

Length of Treatment/Stay

Ten to twelve weeks, depending on patient's response.

Costs

Four weeks of therapy: $5,000.
Each subsequent week: $500.
Medication to take home: $50 per week ($1,300 for six months).
Apartment rentals: $650 to $1,000 per month.
Food: approximately $700 per month.

Method of Payment

Cash (in United States dollars), traveler's checks, and cashier's checks are accepted. Some insurance companies will reimburse.

Institute of Applied Biology

26 East 36th Street
New York, New York 10015
United States

(212) 685–0111

Contact Person

Elena Avram.

Primary Personnel

Emanuel Revici, M.D.; Bijan Kosbin, M.D.

Directions

Located in Manhattan on the East Side. Easily accessible by car and public transportation.

Background

Dr. Revici's treatments have been in evolution since the mid-1920s. His therapy is an outgrowth of his studies on lipids and their role in physiopathology. The agents are derived from natural sources or are synthesized to act like natural substances in the body. They are either lipidic or lipid-based and may incorporate various elements or metals (which are nontoxic in this form). The basic aim is to correct or control disorders in the body's defense systems.

The institute is outpatient only. There is no X-ray or CAT scan equipment on the premises, but those procedures are prescribed. Blood chemistries are also prescribed, although the actual analysis is done by outside labs. Urine samples and some blood samples are analyzed at the institute.

Illness Treated

Dr. Revici has had some success with every type of cancer, even at late stages. The most spectacular cases appear to be long-term remissions in brain, lung, pancreatic, and metastasized breast carcinoma. The institute also treats virtually all degenerative diseases, as well as AIDS.

Treatment Offered

Nontoxic chemotherapy, developed by Dr. Revici through original research over a period spanning nearly seven decades. The treatment is administered either orally, through drops in capsules, or by injection. The treatment is individually guided. The response seems to be individual.

Related Readings

Research in Physiopathology as Basis of Guided Chemotherapy With Special Application to Cancer by Emanuel Revici, M.D. Princeton, New Jersey: Van Nostrand Company Inc., 1961.

Emanuel Revici, M.D.: A Review of His Scientific Work by Dwight L. McKee, M.D., editor. Institute of Applied Biology, 1985.

Individuals interested in obtaining other publications by or about Dr. Revici should write to the institute.

Length of Treatment/Stay

Variable, depending on stage of illness. The frequency of visits often is irregular. Most of the time, the patient, following Dr. Revici's instructions and keeping in touch by phone (no charge), administers the treatment at home.

Costs

First consultation, with treatment: $500.
Repeat visits: $95.
Medicare: $65, including medicine.
Some simple procedures: $50.

Method of Payment

Cash and personal checks are accepted. Insurance companies have been honoring reimbursement requests on the whole. Medicare is accepted, but not Medicaid. No assignments. For individuals who can prove financial need, arrangements may be made. Medication is free. Donations for medicine are welcome (and vital to meet operating expenses).

Instituto Cientifico de Regeneración, S.A.

Calle Ensenada #393
Col. Cacho
Tijuana, B.C.
Mexico

011–52–66–849231
011–52–66–849237

United States Address:
I.C.D.R.
Suite 104
2310 Via Tercero
San Ysidro, California 92073
United States

Fax: (213) 516–6735

Contact Person

Jean Hesse, a former cancer patient of the institute. Write to her at P.O. Box 503, Gardena, California 90247 or phone (213) 538–3277.

Primary Personnel

Neil Norton, M.D. (diagnostic research).

Directions

After crossing the international border, proceed onto bridge under overpass. Remain in right lane while crossing the bridge. Make no left turns. After crossing bridge, turn right at first traffic circle and get into left lane immediately. In a very short distance is another traffic circle. Proceed through this circle without turning, staying to the left. At the first traffic signal turn left. Go one block and turn left again. Continue across a major intersection (Aqua Caliente). Continue up the street (Calle Ensenada) until you reach the institute. It is on your left near the end of the block. It is a large two-story building with a brown cement-block wall on one side of the walkway and a rock wall on the other. At the front of the second story is a large mural. There are no street signs.

Background

Dr. Norton is licensed by the Mexican Government. He has been practicing for 40 years. The strictly outpatient clinic has what it calls a urine probability analysis, which uses computer instrumentation to obtain information quickly from the processed specimen. The analysis will indicate various pathological problems, their locations, and a comprehensive diagnosis.

Also used in diagnosis and treatment are certain heat and electronic procedures, many of which originated in other parts of the world and some of which were developed at the institute. A Symcomp computer analysis uses a list of the patient's symptoms and the results of the patient's lab tests to produce complex explanations for the primary cause of a patient's illness.

Illness Treated

Cancer, all degenerative conditions, arthritis, herpes, tuberculosis, diabetes, and multiple sclerosis.

Treatment Offered

Intravenous with oral support, intramuscular injections, and whatever other oral medications are indicated by the computer testing. Heat and electronic procedures are also involved.

Related Readings

Audio tapes of Dr. Norton's lectures are available for a fee.

Length of Treatment/Stay

One week of treatment (including testing and consultations), followed by one week of rest. This pattern is repeated as needed.

Costs

Consultation (six months): $150.
Lab work (as needed): $250 to $600.
Treatment: Depends on medication involved, but the daily average is $125.
Urine probability analysis: $50 to $75.

Method of Payment

A deposit of $1,000 is required before treatment and lab tests are begun. Any balance is to be paid upon leaving each week. Traveler's checks, cash, and personal checks are accepted. Most insurance is applicable.

Internal and Preventive Medical Clinic

6565 De Moss, Suite 202
Houston, Texas 77074
United States

(713) 981–7500

Primary Personnel

Owen Robins, M.D.

Background

This is a total health care program designed to give "knowledge to help ourselves in all phases" of health. The program considers spiritual factors, mental factors, physical factors (diet and exercise), and environmental factors when dealing with an illness. It emphasizes doing all things with love to attempt to get the individual into a better state of health.

Illness Treated

Cancer and a general range of illnesses.

Treatment Offered

Metabolic treatment is used in relationship to the clinic's general philosophy. The basic program is 24 months long. It starts with tests and medical history; a physical exam includes ECG, blood tests, proctosigmoidoscopic exam, and (for women) a pelvic exam and pap smear. Patients are sent home with an FEC test for detection of occult blood in the stools. Other tests may be indicated. Specific directions for preparation of the tests will be given through the clinic.

Four days later, the patient returns for analysis and interpretation of the lab reports. Other follow-up visits are scheduled.

The clinic has outpatient facilities only.

Length of Treatment/Stay

Treatment continues for 24 months. The initial workup takes seven days.

Costs

Office visits cost $96 per hour. The initial office visit lasts approximately one hour. Diagnostic tests are $500–$550 for men and $550–$600 for women. Phone calls longer than three minutes cost $10 and up.

Method of Payment

Cash only. Payment is due in cash when the services are rendered.

International Medical Center

16 de Septiembre #2215
3203–Cd. Juarez
Mexico

0115216–16–26–01

United States Office:
424 Executive Center Boulevard, Suite 100
El Paso, Texas 79902

(800) 621–8924
(915) 534–0272

Patient Residence:
Hotel Plaza
Ave. Lincoln Y Coyoacan
Cd. Juarez, Chih.
Mexico

0115216 13–13–10
0115216 13–20–78

Primary Personnel

Francisco Soto, M.D., medical director; Ricardo James, M.D., assistant medical director; Bill Carson, U.S. director.

Directions

Patients use El Paso International Airport, El Paso Greyhound bus station, or Amtrak station, and are transported to and from the clinic. The clinic is located ten minutes from downtown El Paso, Texas.

Background

This clinic was started as Clinica Paso del Norte, basically a cancer clinic until September 1989, when H. Ray Evers, M.D., and Francisco Soto, M.D., brought all their talents and protocols to the clinic so that it now treats, in addition to cancer, all forms of chronic degenerative disease.

Illness Treated

Cancer, heart disease, circulatory problems, arthritis, diabetes, amyotrophic lateral sclerosis (Lou Gehrig's disease), chronic fatigue syndrome, Epstein Barr virus, candidiasis, hypoglycemia, Parkinson's disease, Alzheimer's disease, and any other degenerative disease.

Treatment Offered

Chelation, hyperbaric oxygen, electrotherapy, hydrotherapy, colon therapy, ozone therapy, detoxification, respiratory therapy, physical therapy, acupuncture, chiropractic services, cartilage (shark and bovine), Koch vaccine, enzyme and nutritional therapy, and a multi-therapeutic approach with live cell therapies.

Length of Treatment/Stay

Three to four weeks recommended.

Costs

Total cost depends on the treatment recommended and therefore varies substantially. But generally, cancer treatment averages $3,500 to $4,000 per week; treatment for other diseases averages $3,000 to $3,500 per week. All prices include room, board, and transportation from El Paso. The price for the live cell therapy depends on the type and number of injections. A three-day detoxification program is available for $700.

Method of Payment

Cashier's checks, money orders, cash, and personal checks are accepted. Visa and Master-Card are accepted in Juarez and discounted at Mexican banks. Payments are due at the beginning of each week. The center is not in a position to rely on insurance payments; some private companies have been paying, although the collection period runs three to six months.

P. Jayalashmi, M.D.

6366 Sherwood Road
Philadelphia, Pennsylvania 19151
United States

(215) 473–4226
(215) 473–7453

Health Retreat:
R.D. #1 Box 148
Lehighton, Pennsylvania 18235
United States

Contact Person

Connie.

Primary Personnel

P. Jayalashmi, M.D.; K.R. Sampathachar, M.D.

Background

Although this center offers limited inpatient facilities—with diagnosis, treatment, and counseling available—it is primarily an outpatient facility. Also offered is a free public lecture series and a free monthly support group with planned agendas on living healthfully.

Also available, two hours from Philadelphia, is the New Life Wholistic Health Retreat. The resort offers treatment for some chronic diseases; aid in stress and weight reduction and in stopping smoking; biofeedback; and allergy tests. Treatments, chelation, colonics, and some diagnostic tests can be done there as well. Other activities are aerobics, boating, health spa, golf, tennis, cycling, classes, yoga, movies, and sightseeing.

Illness Treated

Cancer, allergies, arthritis, hypertension, heart disease, AIDS, and all chronic diseases.

Treatment Offered

Nutrition, stress reduction, chelation, megavitamins, enzymes, allergy control, detoxification, colonic irrigation, trigger point injections, and anti-candida treatment. Some techniques used are thermography, acupuncture, cytotoxic tests, rotation diet, provocative skin testing, neutralization therapy, Simonton's visualization, noninvasive vascular study (an electronic analysis of circulation), hair analysis, and iridology. This therapy has been practiced for eight years.

Related Readings

Yeast Syndrome by Dr. Trowbridge.

The center will furnish upon request information regarding past patients.

Length of Treatment/Stay

Ranges from one weekend to a couple of months.

Costs

The initial consultation is $60. Lab tests and X-rays are extra. Fees for services are usually a few hundred dollars.

Method of Payment

Cash, checks, Visa, and private insurance are accepted for medical tests.

Laboratory Atlanta

203 B Medical Way
Riverdale, Georgia 30274
United States

(404) 991–1971

Primary Personnel

Kenneth Alonso, M.D., F.A.C.P., F.C.A.P.

Directions

Located near Hartsfield International Airport.

Background

Dr. Alonso is a clinical professor of pathology at Morehouse School of Medicine and considers himself a pioneer in the biological therapy of cancer. The center is an outpatient facility.

Illness Treated

Cancer and immune disorders.

Treatment Offered

Continuous infusion chemotherapy, immunotherapy with interferon and interleukin-2, human monoclonal antibody therapy, and radioiodine. Therapy is guided by human tumor stem cell assay (anti-cancer agents are placed in tissue culture to choose only those that may work in the patient).

Fresh tumor is cloned and examined for sensitivity to radiation, heat, drugs, interferon, cytokines, and other agents. Based on the stem cell assay, a chemotherapy regimen is developed that employs continuous infusion of appropriate agents in low doses for extended time periods. Radiation and heat are employed locally as indicated by the stem cell assay. Monoclonal antibody is raised to patient's tumor at the time of initial cloning. Therapy is tailored for outpatient treatment. Cytokines and antibodies are considered only when maximal tumor burden reductions have been achieved. Antibodies are employed only as carrier for radioisotope for therapy. When appropriate, tumor necrosis factor and interleukin-2 are used.

Related Readings

Dr. Alonso has published many books and articles. Curriculum vita is available on request.

Length of Treatment/Stay

Varies. Stem cell assay requires fresh tissue from biopsy; this may be flown in from anywhere around the world overnight.

Costs

Initial evaluation and consultation: $150.
Stem cell assay: $800.
Monoclonal antibody: $12,000.

Method of Payment

Insurance, bank cards, cash, and checks are accepted.

Livingston Foundation Medical Center

3232 Duke Street
San Diego, California 92110
United States

(619) 224–3515
Fax: (619) 224–6253

Contact Person

Patricia Huntley, director.

Primary Personnel

Kenneth C. Forror, M.D.

Directions

Exit Sea World offramp from Highway 5, or take Rosecrans to Midway and Duke Street.

Background

Livingston Foundation Medical Center was established in 1969 by the late Virginia C. Livingston, M.D., an internationally recognized clinician, healer, and medical researcher who devoted her life to the study of the body's immune system and its relationship to human diseases.

Today, the medical center provides the latest immunological treatment programs based upon the models developed by Dr. Livingston during her more than 50 years of research. The modern, well-maintained facility includes on-site clinical laboratories, a complete nutritional kitchen, and examination and meeting rooms.

The medical center treats people on an outpatient basis. It does not accept patients requiring bed care, though it will provide advice and guidance on the home-application of specific treatments for non-ambulatory or bedridden patients.

Illness Treated

Potentially life-threatening diseases, such as lupus, arthritis, cancer, and scleroderma; also less-serious conditions, such as allergies and stress-induced syndromes. The center offers a preventive program, too.

Treatment Offered

Strengthening the body's immune system with vaccines, diet and nutrition, vitamins, psychological counseling, detoxification, antibiotics, and traditional drug therapy (as long as it does not damage or suppress the natural immune system).

Related Readings

Food Alive (a cookbook).

Conquest of Cancer: Vaccines and Diet by Virginia Livingston-Wheeler, M.D., with Edmond G. Addeo. Franklin Watts Publishing, 1984. (Patients are encouraged to read this before going for treatments.)

Cancer, A New Breakthrough by Virginia Livingston-Wheeler, M.D.

The center will also furnish upon request information regarding past patients.

Length of Treatment/Stay

Ten days (Monday–Friday for two straight weeks).

Costs

Initial consultation for new patients is free. The estimated cost of the full treatment program is $5,500 for ten days. The estimated cost of the preventive program is $1,200. Living expenses are not included. A detailed information packet is available upon request.

Method of Payment

Insurance may or may not cover fees, for which the patients are financially responsible. Cash, personal checks, traveler's checks, money orders, MasterCard, and Visa are accepted.

Lost Horizon Health Awareness Center

P.O. Box 550
1325 Shangri-La Lane
Oviedo, Florida 32765
United States

(407) 365–6681
Fax: (407) 365–1834

Contact Person

Elizabeth.

Primary Personnel

Roy B. Kupsinel, M.D.

Directions

From I-4, exit at Longwood, Florida, and proceed east on Highway 434 for 12 miles to Shangri-La Lane.

Background

Dr. Kupsinel's approach is holistic. He deals with the entire being: physical, mental, emotional, and spiritual. His emphasis is not on treating the disease but on treating the person who may have various health problems.

Illness Treated

Cancer and other degenerative illnesses.

Treatment Offered

Nutrition, diet, supplements, positive thinking, exercise, and other modalities.

Costs

Costs not submitted for publication.

Manner Clinic

(formerly Cydel Hospital)
Tijuana
Mexico

011–526–680–4422

Mailing Address:
Manner Clinic
P.O. Box 434290
San Ysidro, California 92143–4290
United States

Public Relations:

(800) 433–4962 (Nadine)
(501) 675–4962

Metabolic Research Foundation:

011–526–680–4222

Primary Personnel

Gilberto Alvarez, M.D., senior medical officer.

Directions

Clinic is in Tijuana in the direction of Playas and Ensenada. Please call for specific directions.

Background

This is an inpatient facility with room for 40 patients and one companion each. The accommodations include a suite with twin beds, private bathroom, sitting room, color television, and private phone. Free transportation is available between San Diego airport and the clinic. There is a spa facility on the premises. The clinic, over ten years old, had been run for six years by the late Dr. Manner. The clinic specializes in malignant and nonmalignant degenerative diseases using nontoxic therapies. Bring all your medical records (X-rays, surgery and pathology reports) with you.

Illness Treated

Cancer, arthritis, multiple sclerosis, and other degenerative diseases.

Treatment Offered

Metabolic, cellular, and preventive. Metabolic program includes detoxification, counseling, laetrile, diet, vitamins, minerals, a daily "Manner Cocktail" (9 grams laetrile, 10 cc DMSO, 25 grams vitamin C), emulsified vitamin A, immunostimulants, proteolytic enzymes, biofeedback, coffee detox enemas, whirlpool baths and massages, and in some cases nuclear medicine.

Related Readings

The Death of Cancer by Harold W. Manner. Advanced Century Publishing, 1978.

New Death of Cancer Update. Metabolic Research Foundation, 1988.

Mail-order cassette tapes available.

"Manner Clinic and You," a free cassette tape by Harold W. Manner, Ph.D.

The clinic will also furnish upon request information regarding past patients.

Length of Treatment/Stay

Varies, depending on patient's condition.

Costs

A 21-day stay, including room, meals, tests, and treatment, costs $9,750 for cancer patients, $9,425 for arthritis patients, and $7,150 for multiple sclerosis patients. A companion sharing the room is charged $50 per day.

Method of Payment

Major bank credit cards, traveler's checks, money orders, and cash are accepted. No personal checks are accepted. Most insurance companies will reimburse.

Mantell Medical Clinic

General and Family Practice
6505 Mars Road
Evans City, Pennsylvania 16033
United States

(412) 776–5610

Contact Person

Maryanne Woods, office manager.

Primary Personnel

Donald Mantell, M.D.; Wade Boyle, M.D.; John Lanurn, L.P.N.; Evelyn Mancell, colonics therapist; Cheryl Hixon, IV nurse.

Directions

Pennsylvania Turnpike exit 3 (north from Pittsburgh; south from Ohio) to Route 19. North to first light. Right on Route 228. Left onto Dutilh Road. Make first right onto Mars Road.

Background

The facilities are a converted ranch house with two floors and an extensive parking area.

Illness Treated

Cancer, arthritis, allergies, multiple sclerosis, asthma, and musculoskeletal pains.

Treatment Offered

A multifaceted metabolic approach. The major elements of the therapy are: diet, vitamins, minerals, enzymes, herbs, homeopathy, and an IV with DMSO and vitamin C. Ancillary treatments include colonic irrigation, massage therapy, chelation, clinical ecology, neural therapy (for pain), and hydrotherapy.

Related Readings

Crackdown on Cancer With Good Nutrition by Ruth Yale Long. Nutrition Education Association, 1983.

You Don't Have to Die by Harry M. Hoxsey. Joseph C. Carl, 1977.

The Cancer Syndrome by Ralph W. Moss. Grove Press, 1980.

"Colon Hydrotherapy." *The Nutritional Consultant*, May 1986.

DMSO Handbook by Dr. Bruce Halstead.

The Death of Cancer by Harold W. Manner. Advanced Century Publishing, 1978.

The clinic will also furnish upon request information regarding past patients.

Length of Treatment/Stay

This is an outpatient clinic. The patient will have to stay in a motel if from out of town. Intensive treatments at the clinic run from two to four weeks, depending on the severity of the case.

Costs

The first visit costs $310. Of that, $95 is billed to your insurance (if you have appropriate coverage) and $215 is due. The second visit costs $50 plus supplements (one month's supply ranges from $300 to $450). This doesn't include ancillary treatments.

Method of Payment

Cash, checks, MasterCard, and Visa are accepted. Insurance covers diagnostic testing only. Out-of-state residents must pay for diagnostic testing unless covered by Medicare or Blue Shield.

Meadowlark Health Center

26126 Fairview Avenue
Hemet, California 92544
United States

(714) 927–1343

Contact Person

John Chitty.

Primary Personnel

Lawrence H. Taylor, M.D.; Evarts Loomis, M.D.

Directions

Hemet is between Los Angeles and Palm Springs. It is a quiet city at the foot of San Grogonio Mountain.

Background

Meadowlark, California's original holistic health retreat, was founded in 1957. It has adopted Dr. Taylor's new science as the basis for its treatment of life-threatening illnesses:

New Cancer Science	*Old Cancer Science*
1. Detects individual differences.	1. Averages individual differences.
2. Treatment is personalized, even in similar cancers.	2. Similar cancers treated the same.
3. Nontoxic therapies. Treatments support.	3. Selective toxicity. Treatments destructive.
4. Treats the total body.	4. Treats the disease.
5. Integrates body systems into treatment plans.	5. Reductionist theories lead to cytotoxic therapies.
6. Supports optimum nutrition.	6. Generally omits nutritional science.
7. Insists on carcinogen elimination for healing.	7. Views carcinogens as causes but does not relate them to the curing.
8. Relates good emotions to health and bad emotions to illness.	8. Emotions and stresses are not factored into treatment plans.
9. Proves relationships between immune system and emotions.	9. Treatment is generally harmful to parts of the system.
10. Theory: Cancer is a sign or symptom.	10. Theory: Cancer is the disease.
11. Identifies and corrects various pathopsychological problems.	11. Identifies the type and stage of the malignancy.
12. Unlimited treatment options.	12. Treatments limited to surgery, chemotherapy, and radiation.
13. Investigating: mind-body-spirit connections, mineral and vitamin deficiencies in hormone dysregulation, and the effect on the immune system of malabsorption problems.	13. Investigating: biological modifiers, gene function control, viral and cell chromatin, and the regulation of cell division.

Illness Treated

Cancer, arthritis, heart disease, multiple sclerosis, chronic fatigue syndrome, and other serious health problems that have not responded satisfactorily to previous treatment.

Treatment Offered

First, comprehensive examinations, to detect biochemical, hormonal, nutritional, and psychogenic abnormalities. Then testing and other discovery methods, such as endocrine production and targeting organ responses to hormones. Each person requires his own treatment program. In general, however, therapy includes nutrition, detoxification, immune system support, and the development of healing perceptions based upon each person's religious or spiritual background. Chelation therapy is often used.

Length of Treatment/Stay

Six to twelve days.

Costs

Medical treatment varies, but cost for six days can go up to $2,000.

Method of Payment

Upon registration, $1,000 is due, plus 20% of the expected medical charges. Personal checks, traveler's checks, and credit cards are accepted.

Mission Medical Clinic

Playas de Tijuana
B.C.
Mexico

Mailing Address:
4492 Camino de la Plaza
Suite 362
San Ysidro, California 92173
United States

(619) 662–1578

Primary Personnel

James Gunier, H.M.D., Ph.D.; Roberto Diaz, M.D.

Directions

Approximately 15 miles south of San Diego. You may call for exact directions, but patients can stay at the International Motor Inn [(619) 662–1578] in San Ysidro, California, and ride a free shuttle bus to the clinic.

Background

The center, founded in 1983, is an outpatient clinic that uses the European anti-aging cellular revitalization treatment and other support modalities. It claims tumors decrease very rapidly during this program.

Illness Treated

Cancer, tumors, arteriosclerosis, arthritis, stroke, Alzheimer's, Parkinson's, brain dysfunction, memory loss, chronic fatigue, aging problems, and all chronic degenerative diseases.

Treatment Offered

A life-extending, anti-aging program using European live cell, therapeutic immunology, RNA regeneration, GH3, vitamins and minerals administered intravenously, homeopathy, germanium, herbology, Koch vaccine, enzymes, HCl, Rife, chelation, counseling, diet, lifestyle changes, and a personalized follow-up program.

Related Readings

The center will furnish upon request information regarding past patients.

Length of Treatment/Stay

Three weeks of treatment at the clinic is recommended.

Costs

Treatment: $150 to $400 per day, depending on which program the patient chooses.
Follow-up home program (three to four months): $300 to $1,500.

Method of Payment

Cash and traveler's checks are the only methods accepted. Prepayment is required. Most private insurance companies will cover at least a considerable portion of the expenses.

Natural Health Center

P.O. Box N–8941
Third Terrace
Collins Avenue
Nassau
Bahamas

(809) 326–6565
(809) 323–3530
Fax: (809) 322–6606

Contact Person

Petra Ingraham.

Primary Personnel

Michael J. Ingraham, M.D., Ph.D.

Directions

Regular daily flights out of Miami, Florida.

Background

The doctor has a strong background in holistic medicine, German electro-acupuncture diagnostics, bio-energetic medicine, and Mora therapy.

Illness Treated

AIDS, chronic fatigue, selected cancers, and all other chronic degenerative diseases, such as rheumatoid arthritis, diabetes, and coronary heart disease. However, the center usually will not accept patients who have metastatic cancer—especially if they have received chemotherapy.

Treatment Offered

The patient's first visit entails a routine physical, a review of recent blood tests, urine analysis, and hair analysis. The patient will receive an electroacupuncture investigation using the Computron, which determines the therapy and which monitors the treatment daily for effectiveness and to suggest possible changes. Diet and lifestyle changes will be designed on an individual basis. Also, traditional acupuncture and Moxa, Mora therapy, ozone therapy (rectal, vaginal, and intravenous available), magnetic coil therapy, Rife frequencies, live cell injections, intravenous DMSO and hydrogen peroxide, chelation, homeopathic remedies, neural therapy, naturopathic herbals and Chi-Gong therapy, DMSA (oral and parenteral), intravenous vitamins, amino acids, ort-moleculars, chiropractic manipulation, Shiatsu massage, dental testing to remove heavy metals, and galvanic current.

Length of Treatment/Stay

One to two weeks of treatment for most chronic fatigue and other degenerative-type illnesses. Three to six weeks for AIDS and cancer. The center is an outpatient clinic, so patients cannot stay there. Petra can help arrange for your accommodations. Treatments usually start at 9 a.m. and last anywhere from two to five hours. Patients should have a full breakfast before beginning treatment.

Costs

One week of treatment (including the physical, the basic lab tests, the hair and urine analysis, the medication, and the therapy): $2,500.
Three weeks of treatment: $6,500.
Six weeks of treatment: $12,000.
Accommodations cost extra, usually $60 and up per night, but actual price for a room varies according to the season.

Method of Payment

Personal checks and Visa are accepted, but money orders and traveler's checks are preferred. Insurance is accepted, but check with your insurance company first. On the first day, patients will be asked to sign a release form and to make payment in full.

Nevada Clinic

3720 Howard Hughes Parkway
Suite 270
Las Vegas, Nevada 89109
United States

(702) 732–1400
(800) 641–6661

Contact Person

D. Gregory Olson, clinic administrator.

Primary Personnel

F. Fuller Royal, M.D., H.M.D., medical director; Daniel F. Royal, D.O., H.M.D.

Directions

Located one and a half miles north of McCarran International Airport, the clinic is at the northwest corner of Sands and Paradise.

Background

A staff of 30 runs this 10,000-square-foot outpatient clinic. They perform routine blood tests and standard procedures done by other physicians, as well as non-standard procedures. They have electrodiagnostic equipment for measuring abnormal electromagnetic energy fields of the body.

Illness Treated

Cancer; the best responders are liver metastases and colon and breast cancers. Also allergies, arthritis (all types), lupus erythematosus and other collagen diseases, cardiovascular diseases, arteriosclerotic diseases, and AIDS.

Treatment Offered

Homeopathy, chelation, acupuncture, and acuscope.

Length of Treatment/Stay

One to fourteen days. Thirty days for chelation patients.

Costs

The cost for a new patient is $700–$900, which covers the cost of complete evaluation, allergy testing, medication, and treatment for the first day. Return office visits are $55 each day.

Method of Payment

Visa, MasterCard, Discover, Diners Club, cash, and checks are accepted. The clinic will not accept insurance but will help the patient complete the proper forms for reimbursement.

New Hope Naturopathic Medical Center

2525 Roseville Garden Drive, #203
Windsor, Ontario N8T 3J8
Canada

(519) 944–6000

Primary Personnel

Lauri D. Campbell, N.D.

Directions

Located 20 minutes from downtown Detroit, Michigan.

Background

Dr. Campbell received his bachelor's degree from the University of Waterloo in Waterloo, Ontario, and his doctorate from the John Bastyr College of Naturopathic Medicine in Seattle, Washington. He is board certified in general practice by the Ontario Drugless Practitioner's Board, is licensed in Ontario as a doctor of naturopathic medicine, and uses only natural therapies in treating his patients. Dr. Campbell offers food and chemical allergy testing and treatment, nutritional management of chronic degenerative disease, prevention and treatment of cardiovascular disease, orthomolecular nutrition, Candida treatment of premenstrual syndrome, and pain control. New Hope Naturopathic is an outpatient clinic only.

Illness Treated

Those where the immune system has not been destroyed and is capable of responding to natural, nontoxic immune support. Also treats AIDS.

Treatment Offered

Homeopathy, herbs, Koch therapy, germanium therapy, essiac herbal tea, nutritional support, immune system stimulation, orthomolecular medicine, clinical ecology, acupuncture, and visualization therapy.

Length of Treatment/Stay

Two days to four weeks.

Costs

Regular office call (30 minutes): $65.
Brief office call (15 minutes): $35.
Extended office call (beyond 30 minutes): Prorated for additional time spent.
Mariel energy balancing session (30 minutes): $65.
Orthomolecular metabolic energy analysis (blood sample): $120.
Food allergy panel (225 foods): $225.
Contact allergy panel: $75.
Individual vitamin and mineral levels: $45.
Urinalysis (nine-check system): $5.
Full degenerative metabolic testing and workup: $950.
Full metabolic workup including orthomolecular blood test, metabolic function blood tests, and special rate assessments and analysis: $950.
Total first office visit, testing, and immune supports: $300–$1,800.

Method of Payment

Visa, MasterCard, cash, and certified checks are accepted. Blue Cross has been reimbursing for the clinic's services and testing.

Open Clinic

1333 Pacific Avenue
Suites E & H
San Francisco, California 94109
United States

(415) 776–0208

Contact Person

Sunny Wong, chief administrator.

Primary Personnel

Lau Koon-Hung, M.D.; Angela Tsai, O.M.D.; Anthony G. Payne, N.D., N.M.Dip., D.Sc.; and Gabriele Caluwaert, R.N.

Background

Open Clinic is affiliated with the San Francisco School of Chinese Medicine.

Illness Treated

Chronic cancer.

Treatment Offered

The clinic provides hyperbaric oxygen (HBO) therapy; traditional Chinese medical treatments; various naturopathic modalities; and adjunctive cancer care, using Dr. Payne's biochemical approach of anti-proliferation/cytodifferentiation therapy, immunopotentiation therapy, and anti-neoplastic support.

Related Readings

Naturopathic Medicine: A Question and Answer Primer for Laypersons. San Francisco School of Chinese Medicine Press, 1990.

Dr. Payne writes a health column for the *National Educator*. His writings have also appeared in *Whole Foods, Health Consciousness, Holistic Hotline* (newsletter of the American Nutritional Medical Association), *Mensa Bulletin,* and other publications. The clinic has available a 26-page monograph by Dr. Payne on his adjunctive cancer therapy, written for scientifically literate lay persons.

Costs

Costs not submitted for publication.

Method of Payment

Most therapies require prepayment. Payment plans are available in some cases. Hyperbaric oxygen therapy is recognized by many insurance carriers. The clinic will help in filing claim forms.

James R. Privitera, M.D.

105 North Grandview Avenue
Covina, California 91723
United States

(818) 966–1618

Background

This is a nutrition and allergy office, although patients with other diseases, including cancer, go for whole body treatment. Dr. Privitera is a consulting physician, not a family physician, and has had this practice for more than 15 years. His nurses screen calls and explain the program to those who are interested. As a result of a problem he had in treating cancer patients using laetrile, a cancer patient must bring all records and understand that the doctor does not treat cancer as such. Dr. Privitera sees patients with other holistic physicians in other countries such as Mexico and Germany. He keeps up with the latest therapies throughout the world.

Illness Treated

All diseases.

Treatment Offered

Nutritional and immunological enhancement.

Length of Treatment/Stay

Three weeks.

Costs

A $4 fee is charged for processing insurance forms. Check with the office for other fees, which were not submitted for publication.

Method of Payment

MasterCard and Visa are accepted. MediCal stickers are not accepted. Insurance is accepted.

Program for Studies of Alternative Medicines

(Programa de Estudios de Medicinas Alternativas)

Centro de Educacion Continua y Abierta
Universidad de Guadalajara
Calle Escuela Militar de Aviacion #16
Sector Hidalgo
Gualajara, Jal.
Mexico

(36) 166155, (36) 157395, (36) 301094, (36) 300085, or (36) 300934.
Fax: (36) 370030 or (36) 193722.

Primary Personnel

Hector E. Solorzan, M.D., Ph.D., director.

Directions

Guadalajara, the second largest city in Mexico, is accessible by plane, car, and train.

Background

The University of Guadalajara's Program for Studies of Alternative Medicines was established in 1985. Its goal is to investigate, teach, and spread the qualified use of alternative medicines. A seminar is usually held each month on a particular alternative medicine. Some of the seminars are for lay people who want to learn how to prevent disease. Patients who are already sick can be taught how to help the body heal itself.

The school also offers two post-graduate courses on alternative medicines. One is on acupuncture.

Illness Treated

All chronic degenerative diseases, such as cancer, arthritis, lupus, AIDS, diabetes, migraine, multiple sclerosis, allergies, etc.

Treatment Offered

Approximately 216 different alternative therapies, including DMSO, chelation therapy with EDTA, shark cartilage, homeopathy, acupuncture, moxibustion, laser acupuncture, biofeedback, trace minerals, amino acids, electromagnetism, electrolypolisis, massage, cocarboxilase, enzymes, nutrition therapy, magadoses of vitamins, colon therapy, live cell therapy, electroacupuncture according to Voll, neural therapy, ear medicine according to Nogier, Vega method, iridology, herbs, and homotoxicology. No single method is a cure-all, so different treatments are combined according to the needs of the patient. Orthodox medicine can also be used, but in small doses.

Length of Treatment/Stay

The more chronic the disease, the longer the stay. The longest stay is three weeks. Then the patient follows the program at home and can return if he wishes.

Costs

Costs not submitted for publication, but the means of the patient are considered.

Vladimir Rizov, M.D.

8311 Shoal Creek Boulevard
Austin, Texas 78758
United States

(512) 451–8149

Primary Personnel

Dr. Vladimir Rizov.

Background

Dr. Rizov does not turn patients away but explains to them what they can realistically expect.

Illness Treated

Cancer; best responder is prostate cancer. He also treats cardiovascular problems, arthritis, allergies, chronic fatigue, fungal infections, and obesity; and he offers an anti-aging program.

Treatment Offered

Laetrile, orally and intravenously, with vitamin C, B complex, and DMSO; EDTA; enzymes; nutritional evaluation and correction; detoxification; chelation; oxygen therapy; and homeopathy.

Related Readings

Cancer and Vitamin C by Ewan Cameron and Linus Pauling. Linus Pauling Institute of Science and Medicine, 1979.

Bypassing Bypass by Elmer Cranton, M.D.

Length of Treatment/Stay

Cancer, six weeks. Other problems, variable length.

Costs

Introductory appointment: Free.
Six weeks of treatment: $7,000.

Method of Payment

Personal checks are accepted. Although the doctor's office will help the patient fill out insurance forms, it's up to the patient to collect reimbursement from the insurance company. Patients pay daily. Those who pay in advance for the full treatment will receive a 10% discount (non-refundable).

Ruscombe Mansion Community Health Center

4801 & 4803 Yellowwood Avenue
Baltimore, Maryland 21209
United States

(301) 367–7300
Fax: (301) 356–6216

Contact Person

Zoh M. Hieronimus, founder and executive director.

Primary Personnel

About 25 practitioners in private practice work independently and/or integratively to address the unique needs of each client.

Directions

Easy access from highway I-83. Call for details or write for brochure.

Background

Founded in 1984, Ruscombe Mansion annually serves approximately 6,000 outpatient clients—children and adults with acute or chronic illness. The center focuses on giving individuals and families healthy life skills in addition to medical and therapeutic support for the recovery and/or maintenance of health. Support groups, educational programs, an organic foods co-op, and other services are offered at the center by Ruscombe and other non-profit organizations in the Baltimore community. The center is located in two historic mansions within an urban townhouse development adjacent to one of Baltimore's older wildlife sanctuaries.

Illness Treated

Ruscombe Mansion practitioners assist in a client's recovery from the common cold, AIDS, cancer, chronic fatigue, emotional issues, learning disabilities, etc.

Treatment Offered

The premise is to address the whole person and not the disease per se. The physical, emotional, mental, and spiritual needs of each client are considered integral to well-being. All illnesses, therefore, are addressed at the center on an individualized basis focusing on non-toxic and noninvasive health care options such as acupuncture (traditional), acupressure massage, anthroposophical medicine, attitudinal healing, Bach flower remedies, biofeedback, chiropractic techniques, craniopathy, dance therapy, family and individual counseling, Feldenkrais movement, general medicine, guided imagery and music, herbal therapy, homeopathic medicine, homeopathic study group, hypnotherapy, massage, music therapy, nutritional counseling, organic foods, Reiki, Rolfing, stress management, study groups and classes, support groups, vegetarian cooking classes, yoga (kirpalu), and zero balancing.

Related Readings

A lending library is available at Ruscombe Mansion. For suggested reading lists, write or call the center.

Length of Treatment/Stay

Appointments are scheduled for weekdays, weekends, and evenings. Most clients reside in the Maryland, Pennsylvania, or Virginia areas and return home after their appointments. Although there are no inpatient accommodations, the center will help facilitate nearby hotel reservations.

Costs

Fees range from $35–$175 per hour, depending on the services contracted. Clients must give practitioners at least 24 hours' notice on all appointment cancellations or face additional charges.

Method of Payment

Checks, money orders, and cash are accepted. Insurance is accepted for some services; although many of the health care options are third-party reimburseable, clients should check with their own insurance company first.

Michael B. Schachter, M.D., P.C., and Associates

Two Executive Boulevard
Suite 202
Suffern, New York 10901
United States

(914) 368–4700
Fax: (914) 368–4727

Contact Person

Ask for new-patient educators.

Primary Personnel

Michael Schachter, M.D.; Howard C. Greenspan, D.O.; John J. Reynolds, certified physician's assistant; Sally Minniefield, certified physician's assistant; Dolores Tritico, R.N.

Directions

Less than one minute from exit 14B of the New York State Thruway, the facility is located 30 miles northwest of New York City. LaGuardia Airport in New York and Newark International Airport in New Jersey are each approximately a one-hour car ride from the facility. Kennedy International Airport in New York is an hour and a quarter away by car.

Traveling south: Take the New York Thruway (Route 87), exit at Airmont Road (exit 14B). At end of exit ramp turn left onto Airmont Road, and then at the blinking yellow light turn left again, onto Executive Boulevard. The building is on the right, a little bit past the Holiday Inn (which is on the left). Big green letters on the side of the building spell "Barclay." There is a large parking lot. The office is on the second floor of the four-story building.

Traveling north: Take New York State Thruway (Route 87), exit at Airmont Road (exit 14B). At end of exit ramp turn right onto Airmont Road, then turn left at the blinking yellow light. Proceed as stated above.

Traveling east: Take Route 59 eastward, turn left onto Airmont Road (at the corner is the Ramapo Forum Diner). Turn left at the blinking yellow light and proceed as stated above.

Traveling west: Take Route 59 westward, turn right onto Airmont Road (at the Ramapo Forum Diner), turn left at the blinking yellow light, and proceed as stated above.

Background

The practice, started in 1974 by Dr. Schachter and the late Dr. David Sheinkin, is based on a pragmatic philosophy, combining the best of traditional medicine with alternative or holistic medicine. A variety of alternative treatments are integrated. The emphasis is on education, lifestyle changes, and the patient's taking responsibility for his treatment program by managing it on a partnership basis with his health care provider.

This is an outpatient facility only; but in case of emergency, patients can be referred locally for inpatient care. Patients who are on programs with physicians outside the United States (such as Dr. Nieper and the various Mexican clinics) can receive support from Dr. Schachter and his associates.

Illness Treated

Cancer; the best responders are breast, lung, colon, lymphoma, and Hodgkin's disease. The center also treats AIDS, cardiovascular disorders, arthritis, allergies, Candida-related complex, chronic fatigue syndrome, immune dysfunction, glandular disturbances, psychiatric disorders, neurological conditions, childhood disorders, gastro-intestinal disorders, gynecological disorders, musculoskeletal disorders, and patients who simply want a preventive health care program.

Treatment Offered

First, a complete medical history is taken; then there is a complete physical examination; that's followed by laboratory studies, which include routine blood and urine tests, special cancer markers, nutrient status assessment, an immune profile, and, when indicated, allergy testing. Nutritional and metabolic therapies are then used. Available therapies include ortho-molecular medicine and psychiatry, psychotherapy, clinical ecology, preventive medicine, education, detoxification procedures, diet, nutritional supplements, exercise, stress management, amygdalin, and chelation therapy. Emphasis is on injectable programs: intravenous vitamin C and germanium, amygdalin, DMSO, intravenous hydrogen peroxide, subcutaneous SPL, and intramuscular crude liver. Also, individualized oral supplements, hydrazine sulfate, classical homeopathy, complex homeopathy, biomagnetic field therapy, therapeutic massage, saunas, bowel cleansing, and coffee enemas. Most supplements and other therapeutic devices can be purchased at the facility. Side effects are generally minimal. Work is also done with patients who are on chemotherapy under the care of other physicians.

Related Readings

Unconventional Cancer Treatments. U.S. Congress Office of Technology Assessment, September 1990.

Love, Medicine, and Miracles by Bernie Siegel, M.D. Harper & Row, 1986.

Cancer and its Nutritional Therapies by Dr. Richard Passwater. Keats Publishing (revised edition), 1983.

International Protocols for Individualized, Integrated Metabolic Programs in Cancer Management by Robert W. Bradford, Michael Culbert, and Henry W. Allen. Robert W. Bradford Foundation,

1981.

The Cancer Industry: Unraveling the Politics by Ralph W. Moss. Paragon House, 1989.

Oxygen Therapies by Ed McCabe. Energy Publications, 1988.

Biomagnetic Handbook by William H. Philpott, M.D., and Sharon Taplin. EnviroTech Products, 1990.

The Cancer Survivors by Judith Glassman. Dial Press, 1983.

The Metabolic Management of Cancer by Robert W. Bradford and Michael Culbert. Robert W. Bradford Foundation, 1979.

Length of Treatment/Stay

Two to three weeks for out-of-towners; locals (people from New York, New Jersey, or Connecticut) are seen regularly and followed up indefinitely.

Costs

Three weeks (without room and board): $1,500 to $3,000 for workup, counseling, and injectables program. Oral supplements: $50 to $400 per month; more occasionally.

Method of Payment

Cash, checks, money orders, and credit cards are accepted. The staff will help patients get third-party reimbursements but will not bill third-party insurers directly.

Schafer's Health Centre Ltd.

Box 251
Unity, Saskatchewan S0K 4L0
Canada

(306) 228–2512
Fax: (306) 228–4433

Primary Personnel

Dr. Sir Leo J. Schafer, M.H., R.H.C., L.C.S.P.

Directions

Corner of Highway 14 and Highway 21.

Background

After a prolonged illness, Schafer began studying the natural way of healing. He has read many books and attended many seminars and classes regarding reflexology, massage, iridology, herbology, magnetic therapy, color therapy, music and sound therapy, and radionics analysis. He received an honorary doctor's degree in homeopathy in 1984, and in 1985 he received his doctor's of medicine in holistic healing. On January 5, 1987, he became the 17th recipient of the Dag Hammarskjold award, and on August 30 that same year he was received into the order of the Royal Knights of Justice and given the title "Dr. Sir."

Illness Treated

Cancer and other diseases, including AIDS.

Treatment Offered

Herbology, color therapy, magnet therapy, music and sound therapy, diet and nutrition. Dr. Schafer has over 220 of his own herbal formulas. Treatments may involve use of the Rife functional generator, which he makes and sells. He has been using these therapies for 20 years. There are few, if any, possible side effects.

Length of Treatment/Stay

One hour. This is an outpatient facility.

Costs

Consultation: $35 (plus tax).
Program: $50 to $400 (plus tax).

Method of Payment

Visa, cash, and certified checks are accepted.

Shealy Institute for Comprehensive Health Care

1328 East Evergreen
Springfield, Missouri 65803
United States

(417) 865–5940

Contact Person

C. Norman Shealy, M.D., Ph.D.

Primary Personnel

C. Norman Shealy, M.D., Ph.D.; Roger K. Cady, M.D.; Kenneth L. Everett, R.N.; Kathleen Farmer, Psy.D.; Diane Veehoff, R.N., M.S.W.

Directions

South of highway I-44, in north Springfield, Missouri.

Background

The institute began in 1971 as the first comprehensive pain clinic in the country. It has expanded to include comprehensive health care of all kinds. It has a multidisciplinary team with a staff of 28 highly dedicated, holistically oriented individuals. Their philosophy is to apply all conceivable, safe approaches. Traditional approaches are used when appropriate. The institute provides treatment programs up to eight hours per day for up to 20 patients.

Illness Treated

All illnesses except acute psychosis. These do include cancer. Contact the center to find out the location of its AIDS treatment center.

Treatment Offered

Biogenics, individual counseling, massage, nutritional counseling, biofeedback training, acupuncture, consultations, drug detoxification, electrosleep therapy, facet rhizotomy, nerve blocks, Sarapin injections, smoking control, transcutaneous electrical nerve stimulation, and musical vibration for deep relaxation.

Related Readings

Creation of Health by C. Norman Shealy, M.D., Ph.D., and Caroline Myss, M.A.

90 Days to Self-Help by C. Norman Shealy, M.D. Second edition, 1987.

The Pain Game by C. Norman Shealy, M.D. 1976.

Holos Practice Reports—a monthly newsletter. C. Norman Shealy, M.D., editor.

Length of Treatment/Stay

Fifteen days for most chronic problems; sometimes shorter, and occasionally longer.

Costs

Approximately $4,000 for two weeks of therapy.

Method of Payment

Cash, checks, money orders, and credit cards are accepted. The institute will assist patients in filing insurance, but it does not take insurance assignments.

Sierra Clinic Inc.

30003 Gobernador Logo, Suite 202
Tujuana, B.C.
Mexico

011–52–66–864672

Appointments, Reservations, or *Details*:
P.O. Box 3177
Walnut Creek, California 94598
United States

(415) 935–0162

Contact Person

Mrs. Rory Dominguez.

Primary Personnel

G.J. Palafox, M.D.

Directions

Directions are given at the International Motor Inn, 190 Calle Primero, San Ysidro, California, United States.

Background

Sierra Clinic is operated by Dr. Palafox, who has been practicing in Tijuana for more than 23 years. Dr. Palafox was also managing director of a Catholic nun's hospital in Tijuana for more than 17 years. In the past seven years, he has treated hundreds of terminal and nonterminal cancer patients.

The clinic admits only ambulatory patients into its three-week treatment. These treatments are nontoxic and are said to have no side effects or after-effects. After treatment, the patients are given instructions to help them maintain their immune systems at optimum levels.

After a complete medical history has been taken and a medical exam has been completed, the patients can arrive any day of the week and start treatment the following day, except on Sundays. During treatment, many patients stay in San Ysidro at the International Motor Inn, which provides transportation to the clinic and back. Departure for the clinic is usually at 10:30 a.m., and the patient is back at the inn at about 1 p.m. The patient is then free until the next morning.

Illness Treated

Cancer and senility. Also offers a rejuvenation program.

Treatment Offered

A homeopathic detoxification program, chelation, amino acid supplementation (L-Arginine), thymus extract therapy, and daily injections of vitamins and minerals.

Dr. Palafox also uses Niehans therapy, which consists of live cell injections as the basis of a five-day treatment. The procedure was developed by Dr. Paul Niehans in Switzerland in 1931 as a means of relieving symptoms of senility.

The Niehans therapy for senility includes a complete physical exam, the Niehans cell therapy protocol, and laboratory work, including a complete blood count with differential as well as complete amino acid analysis.

Length of Treatment/Stay

Eighteen days, or eighteen injections.

Costs

Cancer treatment: $3,500, which includes medication and six months of home maintenance. Niehans therapy: $2,300.

Method of Payment

Cashier's checks, approved personal checks, money orders, and credit cards are accepted. Payment must be made when services are rendered.

Valley Cancer Institute

12099 West Washington Boulevard
Suite 304
Los Angeles, California 90066
United States

(213) 398–0013
(800) 488–1370
Fax: (213) 398–4470

Contact Person

Leslie Ralston, director of education.

Primary Personnel

James Bicher, M.D., medical director.

Directions

Take the 405 freeway south to the Culver/Braddock exit or north to the Washington Boulevard exit.

Background

Founded in 1985, the institute specializes in hyperthermic oncology (the use of locally applied heat to destroy tumors). Valley Cancer contains the most advanced hyperthermic technology equipment, including a linear accelerator for radiation therapy. It also has research laboratories and both inpatient and outpatient treatment facilities.

Illness Treated

Cancer, including adenocarcinoma, carcinoma, melanoma, thymoma, squamous cell carcinoma, mesothelioma, sarcoma, lymphoma, basal cell cancer, skin cancer, Kaposi's sarcoma (including AIDS-related), and BPH benign prostate hyperplasia. Effective treatable sites include the brain, bones, throat, thyroid, lungs, breast, liver, pancreas, colon, ovaries, uterus, prostate, and other anatomical sites.

Treatment Offered

Hyperthermia. The treatment is basically nontoxic, reduces pain, and lessens the side effects from standard treatments. The institute also provides nutritional information and educational support.

Related Readings

Dr. Bicher has written eight books and more than 230 articles in professional medical and engineering journals. Call the institute for exact titles.

Length of Treatment/Stay

Varies from patient to patient, but a typical treatment lasts five weeks, five days per week, one hour per day.

Costs

Costs, not submitted for publication, will vary depending on the extent of the cancer and the number of fields of treatment required.

Vital-Life Institute

P.O. Box 294
Encinitas, California 92024
United States

(619) 943–8485
(800) 473–8485
Fax: (619) 436–9642

Contact Person

Patty Harper.

Primary Personnel

Steven R. Schechter, N.D., Ph.D.

Directions

The institute is near highway I-5, along the ocean, between La Costa Avenue and Leucadia Boulevard, 30 minutes north of San Diego Airport, and one hour south of Anaheim.

Background

Dr. Schechter is the author of a book on natural remedies that strengthen the immune system; detoxify the body from chemical pollutants, radiation, X-rays, drugs, and alcohol; generate maximum vitality and health; and prevent or treat disease—including cancer.

Dr. Schechter has been the featured speaker at health industry trade conventions and consumer health expos. He was director of clinical nutrition and medical herbology at a large medical detoxification clinic.

Vital-Life is open Monday–Friday from 9 a.m. to 5 p.m. Health consultations are offered in person, on an outpatient basis, or over the telephone. All information is based on extensive clinical experience and upon thousands of primary scientific research studies documenting the safety and effectiveness of the specific natural remedies.

Illness Treated

Cancers, including breast, lung, liver, lymph, pancreas, colon, cervix, uterus, and prostate; tumors, including brain tumors; AIDS and CIFIDS; Epstein Barr virus; yeast infection; liver-related disorders; environmental injury; and other disorders related to immune deficiency.

Treatment Offered

Therapeutic foods, herbs, vitamin and mineral supplements, amino acids, glandular extracts, enzymes, periodic short fasts, exercise programs, positive visualizations, and other natural remedies.

Related Readings

Fighting Radiation & Chemical Pollutants with Foods, Herbs, & Vitamins: Documented Natural Remedies that Boost Your Immunity & Detoxify by Steven R. Schechter, N.D.

Length of Treatment/Stay

Most treatments on outpatient basis or over the telephone. People may call for a telephone consultation or come to Vital-Life and stay at a nearby hotel or motel.

Costs

Consultation fee: $95 per hour.

Method of Payment

Check, cash, money orders, Visa, and MasterCard are accepted. Some insurance companies will reimburse the client.

Waisbren Clinic

2315 North Lake Drive
Room 815, Seton Tower
Milwaukee, Wisconsin 53211
United States

(414) 272–1929

Contact Person

Ms. Jury, clinic manager.

Primary Personnel

Burton A. Waisbren Sr., M.D., F.A.C.P.

Directions

East of Highway 43 on North Avenue to Lake Michigan. Seton Tower is easily visible.

Background

This therapy is to be used in conjunction with orthodox methods of cancer therapy. Patients can be hospitalized at St. Mary's. The clinic will gladly explain its approach to your personal physician so that you can receive his evaluation before deciding whether to undergo the treatment.

Illness Treated

Cancer; the best responders are lymphoma and lung. Also multiple sclerosis.

Treatment Offered

Mixed bacterial vaccine, Coley-type vaccine transfer factor, BCG, and lymphoblastoid lymphocytes. Sometimes, the clinic will make an autologous vaccine from the patient's tumor cells, and sometimes it will make tumorcidal cultures from the tumor-associated lymphocytes. Fever can be a side effect of the treatment.

Length of Treatment/Stay

One week for evaluations; treatment is usually weekly for four weeks, then monthly.

Costs

One year: $3,000 to $8,000. When attempted, tumor vaccines and tumor-associated lymphocyte cultures are done on a cost-plus basis.

Method of Payment

Cash, bank cards, and American Express are accepted. Any money received from insurance is refunded to the patient.

Warren's Clinic

5121 Evangeline Street
Baton Rouge, Louisiana 70805
United States

(504) 355–3741

Primary Personnel

J.D. Warren, D.C., N.D.

Directions

Five blocks off of Airline Highway.

Background

Dr. Warren has been at this facility for 10 years and has been practicing his therapy for 15 years.

Illness Treated

Cancer; the best responders are lung and colon. Also degenerative diseases, including AIDS.

Treatment Offered

Nutritional and chiropractic, including colonic.

Related Readings

The clinic will provide upon request information regarding past patients.

Costs

No one has exceeded $2,000.

Treatment Centers

Hospitals, Clinics, Physicians, Health Practitioners

Overseas (Australia, Germany, Greece, Japan, Netherlands, New Zealand, Philippines, Spain, Switzerland, United Kingdom)

Auchenkyle

Southwoods Road
Troon, Ayrshire
Scotland
United Kingdom

(0292) 311414

Primary Personnel

Dr. Jan de Vries, D.O., Ph.D., N.D.

Directions

Near Prestwick Airport.

Background

Dr. de Vries has worked with alternative medicine for 26 years and is now operating a versatile center designed to promote wellness. A variety of special programs are available, such as a slimming center (to lose weight via acupuncture), a skin care clinic, and a well woman clinic.

Illness Treated

Most common cancers, multiple sclerosis, arthritis, and AIDS.

Treatment Offered

Naturopathic therapies, including acupuncture, osteopathy, homeopathy, herbal medicine, Kirlian photography, iridology, diapulse, X-rays, physiotherapy, and diet. There are no known side effects from the treatment.

Related Readings

By Appointment Only. Edinburgh: Mainstream Publishing, 1986.

The clinic will also furnish upon request information regarding past patients.

Length of Treatment/Stay

One week.

Costs

Costs not submitted for publication.

Method of Payment

Cash, insurance (check with insurance company first), and credit cards are accepted.

Bay of Plenty Chelation Clinic

Willow House
14 Willow Street
Tauranga
North Island
New Zealand

64–075–782–362
Fax: Same as telephone number.

Primary Personnel

Mike Godfrey, M.B.B.S.

Background

The clinic specializes in environmental and preventive medicine.

Illness Treated

Cancer, Alzheimer's, chronic diseases, and cardiovascular disorders.

Treatment Offered

Nutritional and immunosupportive therapy for chronic diseases and for cancer. Mercury amalgam investigations and safe detoxification protocols. Chelation therapy for cardiovascular disorders and for Alzheimer's disease.

Costs

Costs not submitted for publication.

Bircher-Benner Privatklinik

Kelltenstrasse 48
CH 8044 Zurich
Switzerland

011–41–1251–68–90

Primary Personnel

Werner Portmann, administrative director; H.P. Seiler, M.D.

Background

This inpatient clinic has 70 beds and is set in beautiful surroundings above Zurich. The clinic offers a complete program, including a daily schedule of activities, such as a walk every morning at 7:15, three meals, gymnastics, rest periods, library time, etc.

Bring a medical certificate for hospitalization from your physician.

Illness Treated

Cancer and other degenerative illnesses.

Treatment Offered

Physiotherapy and a special lactovegetarian diet.

Costs

In Swiss Francs (SwF):

Bedridden Patients (including nursing care tax)
Private room: 415–465 SwF per day.
  with bathroom: 505 SwF per day.
Semiprivate room: 365 SwF per day.
  with bathroom: 405 SwF per day.

Other Patients
Private room: 195 SwF per day.
  with bathroom: 255 SwF per day.
Semiprivate room: 175 SwF per day.
  with bathroom: 215 SwF per day.

The approximate weekly costs are 1,500–2,000 SwF in the health division and 3,000–4,000 SwF in the hospital division.

Method of Payment

Cash only is accepted. No credit cards are accepted. Check with your insurance company about coverage.

Bristol Cancer Help Centre

Grove House, Cornwallis Grove
Clifton, Bristol BS8 4PG
England
United Kingdom

011–44–0272–743216 (from the United States)
(0272) 743216 (from England)

Contact Person

Cynthia Slade, administrative director.

Primary Personnel

Gillian Corney, chief executive; Liza Dagnall, therapy administrator.

Directions

By train from London: (Paddington) station to Bristol (Temple Meads). By car from London: M4 westward, M32 into Bristol.

Background

Located in Bristol, one and a half hours due west of London, this was originally opened in 1980 as an outpatient clinic. In 1983, it was relocated and expanded to an inpatient facility. This clinic is not suitable for patients who are nonambulatory or in severe pain.

Illness Treated

Cancer, all types.

Treatment Offered

A program is offered that stimulates the immune system and revitalizes the natural self-healing process. It can be safely used alongside orthodox medical treatment. The therapy is geared to help the whole person: body, mind, and spirit. A wholesome natural diet supplemented by vitamins and minerals, herbal extracts, and Bach flower remedies greatly assists in the self-healing process. Relaxation, meditation, imagery, and visualization calm both body and mind. Individual counseling, art therapy, and spiritual healing harmonize emotions and spirit. Patients are helped to change their orientation and lifestyle. There also is nutritional advice, laying on of hands, creative expression (through movement and sound), and massage. The centre does not profess to offer a cure for cancer; its emphasis is on improving the quality of life.

Related Readings

Loving Medicine by Dr. Rosy Thomson.

Gentle Giants by Penny Brohn. London: Century Publishing.

The Bristol Programme by Penny Brohn.

Length of Treatment/Stay

One day minimum; one week recommended.

Costs

The cost of staying at the centre is 665 pounds per week. This includes all therapy, vitamins, etc. There are no other charges. An accompanying supporter is charged 185 pounds per week. The first one-day visit costs 110 pounds. This covers doctor's visits, meals, and therapy. Return visits cost 25 pounds per day, which includes doctor's visits, meals, etc.

Method of Payment

Visa, Access, checks, cash, and banker's drafts are accepted.

Chronic Disease Control and Treatment Center

Am Reuthlein
D–8675 Bad Steben, den
Germany

011–49–9288/5166
011–49–9267/1702
Fax: 011–49–9267/1040
011–49–9288/7815

Primary Personnel

Dr. Helmut Keller.

Directions

The center is located in northeast Bavaria in the heart of the Franconian Forest.

Background

This facility provides Dr. Keller a place to offer a broad yet individualized therapy dependent on immune monitoring. He continues research into and the application of Carnivora, a standardized phytopharmacon of pressed juices of Dionaea muscipula.

Illness Treated

Cancer, multiple sclerosis, chronic polyarthritis, Crohn's disease, ulcerative colitis, neurodermititis, chronic viral diseases, immune deficiency, and auto-aggressive diseases.

Treatment Offered

Complete immune status evaluation; individualized treatments according to laboratory results and risks; preventative program; program before and after tumor operation designed to prevent metastases; use of copper, zinc, selenium, magnesium, lithium, vitamin C, vitamin E, beta-carotene, ozone therapy, hyperthermia, and continual monitoring during treatment.

Length of Treatment/Stay

Patients are treated Monday through Friday for three to four hours per day. There is a recommended stay of four to six weeks, after which the patient can be released to the referring physician with a suggested treatment schedule.

Costs

Treatment, room, and board for four weeks: 8,000–10,000 deutsche marks.
HIV patients receive Carnivora only; their four-week cost would be 5,000 deutsche marks.

E.D. Danopoulos, M.D.

Rigillis Str. 26 (Private Practice: 12 Rigillis Str.)
106–74 Athens
Greece

011–301–721–5318

Primary Personnel

Prof. E.D. Danopoulos, M.D.

Background

Dr. Danopoulos has a private practice in the heart of Athens, Greece. He works closely with a surgeon who supports his work and who performs any necessary procedures, such as a reversible colostomy for colon cancer patients. The length of stay is approximately two weeks, during which time the patient is monitored and a proper dosage of medication is established.

Illness Treated

Cancer of inner organs, especially liver, colon, skin, and conjunctival.

Treatment Offered

Dr. Danopoulos has found that urea, the crystalloid substance in urine, has intensive anticancer action, particularly with cancer of the liver, colon, skin, lip, and conjunctiva (mucous membrane around the eyeball). The results with colon cancer are encouraging. He has not found any side effects or complications with this therapy. Urea is said to be an inexpensive, nontoxic chemical.

The urea is administered orally, locally, or through colostomy, depending on the location of the tumor. This therapy has been practiced for 17 years.

Related Readings

Dr. Danopoulos has published several articles in the *British Journal of Ophthalmology*, *Lancet*, *Clinical Oncology*, *Ophthalmologica* and the *Journal of Surgical Oncology*.

Length of Treatment/Stay

Two to fifteen days.

Costs

$1,000* if operation is required; $500 for medical care without operation. (Hotel stay, food, etc., not included.)

Method of Payment

Blue Cross-Blue Shield for hospital costs only. Cash is accepted in both American and Greek currencies.

J. Buxalleu Font

Carrer d'Avall No. 44
08350 Arenys de Mar
Spain

(93) 792–0489

Contact Person

J. Buxalleu Font.

Directions

By Car: Arrive at Arenys de Mar from Barcelona from the toll road (direction of Mataro). Keep going straight along highway N-11 to Arenys de Mar. (It is not difficult, because the end of the toll road coincides with highway N-11.)

*=Subject to the value of the U.S. dollar abroad.

By Train: The railway begins at the "cercanias" station in Barcelona and runs along the coast. Arenys de Mar is about 40 kilometers (24 miles) from Barcelona, in the northeast direction.

Background

This is an outpatient clinic only. This therapy has been in use since 1965 without any side effects.

Illness Treated

Cancer only (solid tumors). Sometimes the localization is more important than the type of tumor; liver and brain cancers are difficult.

Treatment Offered

Self-vaccination. The patient's blood is extracted periodically, modified, and injected back into the patient with gammaglobulin. In addition, treatment with a new personal construction molecule has recently begun. It increases immunity while being an antibiotic to malignant cells and nontoxic to normal cells.

Related Readings

A few articles have been published in Spanish journals. The center will provide upon request information regarding past patients.

Length of Treatment/Stay

The minimum length of stay is about three months. The recommended length is indefinite. In three months, with intensive treatment, the metabolic alteration of the organism is curbed. Extending this treatment over several years, the metabolic alteration may be rectified.

Costs

The cost depends on the patient's economic status. The cost of the vaccine together with the complementary treatment is about $600* a month.

*=Subject to the value of the U.S. dollar abroad.

Method of Payment

Cash only is accepted. No insurance or credit cards are accepted.

Holistic Medical Clinic

1–18–11 KY Building 6F
Kita-Oostsuka, Toshima-ku
Tokyo 170
Japan

03–3940–8071
Fax: 03–3917–9753

Contact Person

Tsuneo Kobayashi, M.D., director.

Background

Holistic Medical Clinic is associated with Holistic Tennoudai Clinic and Asia Medical Center. It specializes in preventing cancer and preventing the recurrence of cancer. Its original system for detecting early cancer uses tumor marker combination assay.

Illness Treated

Cancer (all kinds, even advanced stages), cirrhosis of the liver, and chronic hepatitis.

Treatment Offered

Lifestyle improvement advice; refreshment therapy, which cleans the alimentary canal and heightens the immune system; herb medicine (Sun Advance); panax ginseng; vitamins A, C, and E; hair analysis, which leads to suggestions for dietary improvements; hyperthermia; radio frequency therapy; systemic BRM-induced immuno-thermo-chemotherapy; plasma exchange; adoptive sensitized lymphocyte therapy; lymphokine-activated killer cells; and psychosomatic therapy. The actual treatment will depend on the degree of the disease.

Length of Treatment/Stay

Cancer prevention: 1–3 months.
Preventing the recurrence of cancer: 1–3 months.

Advanced cancer: 3–6 months.
Cirrhosis of the liver: 3–4 months.

Costs

Each treatment has a set price in Japanese yen. All references to United States dollars are for the reader's convenience only, are based on one particular day's exchange rates, and are subject to daily fluctuation.
Refreshment therapy: 23,000 yen ($165) per day.
Radio frequency therapy: 50,000 yen ($360) per treatment.
Systemic BRM-induced immuno-thermo-chemotherapy: 100,000 yen ($720) per day.
Sun Advance herb medicine: 54,000 yen ($390) per bottle.
Plasma exchange: 250,000 yen ($1,800) per exchange.
Tumor marker examination test: 80,000–220,000 yen ($570–$1,570).
Adoptive sensitized lymphocyte therapy: 45,000 yen ($320) per treatment.
Lymphokine-activated killer cell therapy: 100,000 yen ($720) per treatment.

Hufeland Klinik for Holistic Immunotherapy

Bismarckstr. 16
D–6990 Bad Mergentheim
Germany

01149 7931 7082

Primary Personnel

Wolfgang Woeppel, M.D., medical superintendent.

Directions

Take a plane to Frankfurt airport. From there, you can catch a train or a taxi for the 90 miles southeast to Bad Mergentheim.

Background

The clinic offers a holistic concept tailored to the individual needs of each patient. The clinic follows the concept that a tumor is only the late-stage symptom of cancer, which is a systemic disease caused by impaired functioning of the body's own defense and repair mechanisms.

Cancer is not merely the disorder of one organ but is an expression of a comprehensive disorder of the whole person in his or her unity of body and soul. Conventional scientific medicine, traditional European naturopathy, and empirical medicine can be selectively used in a way that rebuilds people instead of destroying them. For special questions, call Dr. Woeppel at 01149 7931 44520; the best chances to reach him are on Tuesdays, Thursdays, and Fridays, at 7 p.m. German time (1 p.m. New York time).

Illness Treated

Malignant diseases of all kinds and at all stages, including brain tumors; chronic degenerative diseases, including arthritis, indigestion, and arteriosclerosis; also treats patients who will soon undergo surgery but who first want to strengthen their defenses. Treatment is not possible for acute leukemia, acute infectious diseases, or serious heart conditions. The clinic does not accept patients who are confined to bed. Patients must not be too weak and must be able to walk unaided.

Treatment Offered

Regeneration of the organism by stimulating the detoxifying functions of the liver, kidneys, and intestines with homeopathic medicines, vitamins, minerals, enzymes, multistep oxygen therapy, ozone therapy, and an ovo-lactovegetarian diet; strengthening the body's natural defense mechanisms through active fever therapy, thymus extract, serums, infusions with mistletoe preparations, biological response modifiers, and regeneration of the intestinal flora; psychological treatment to strengthen the patient's will to recover; and, when necessary, careful conventional treatment such as chemotherapy, hormonotherapy, painkillers, etc.

Length of Treatment/Stay

Four to ten weeks, depending on the individual. During the treatment, the patient is adjusted to the therapy, which can be continued at home with the help of a general practitioner. (Although the clinic is usually booked for months ahead of time, it provides for patients to stay at a nearby hotel or in a private accommodation.) It is necessary to bring all documents relating to your illness, such as doctor's reports, laboratory findings, and X-rays.

Costs

Inpatients: $200* per day, which covers board, lodging, medicine, laboratory tests, and doctor's consultations.
Outpatients: $180* per day, which covers medicine, laboratory tests, and doctor's consultations.

*=Subject to the value of the U.S. dollar abroad.

If other medical services are necessary, such as consultations with other specialists, scans, or hospitalization, those who perform the service will bill the patient directly and separately.

Method of Payment

A $4,000* deposit is required upon arrival. Cash and traveler's checks are the only methods accepted. Inquire with your own health insurance company for possible coverage of part or all of the cost of treatment.

Institute for Immunology and Thymus Research

(Institut fur Immunologie und Thymusforschung)
Rudolf–Huch–Str. 14
D–3388 Bad Harzburg
Germany

05322–2033
05322–2034
Fax: 05322–3017

Contact Person

Ingrid Heinze.

Primary Personnel

Milan C. Pesic, M.D.

Directions

Fly to Frankfurt or Hannover airports. Bad Harzburg is approximately a one-hour highway ride from Hannover and approximately three hours from Frankfurt. A train also goes from Hannover to Bad Harzburg.

*=Subject to the value of the U.S. dollar abroad.

Background

THX/Thymex–L, a thymus extract, has been used in the treatment of more than 1.5 million patients in Europe, the United States, and Canada. It is an important immune modulator and immune corrector.

Illness Treated

Cancer; the best responders are lung, bladder, colon, pancreatic, and breast cancer, morbus Hodgkin's, "none" Hodgkin's, and Kaposi's sarcoma. The institute also treats chronic degenerative diseases, including rheumatoid arthritis. Also accepted are patients who have metastatic cancer after having received an operation, radiation therapy, or chemotherapy.

Treatment Offered

THX/Thymex–L. It can be combined with other medicines. A diet is not necessary. After the first injections, it is possible that itching, redness, or swelling can occur locally; that should be treated with ointment. Other side effects are unknown.

It is preferred that the patient first prepare general information about himself, documentation of his illness, and details of the past three treatments received. It is also preferred for the patient to send all the information and medical reports to the institute ahead of time, either by mail or telefax. The office can be telephoned any Thursday from 3–6 p.m. (German time). Full accommodations for the patient and accompanying persons are available at the clinic. The patient will find treatment easier by taking those accommodations, but he may choose instead to stay in one of the hotels in Bad Harzburg.

Related Readings

Experiences and Experimental Results with Whole Thymus Extract THX by Milan C. Pesic, M.D. Thymus Medizinischer Fachbuchverlag, Bad Harzburg, 1986.

"Therapeutic Possibilities of Thymic Preparations" by Milan C. Pesic, M.D. *A New Dimension in Scientific Research*, Vol. 1, No. 5:9–19, Washington.

"THX (Gesamt–Thymus–Extrakt nach Sandberg) bei der primar chronischen Polyarthritis und Gonarthrose" by Milan C. Pesic, M.D. *Erfahrungsheilkunde*, Bd. 31, Heft 10:790–796, Haug Verlag, Heidelberg, 1982.

Thymus—Zentrale der Immunitat und Endokrines Steuerungsorgan by Milan C. Pesic. Haug Verlag, Heidelberg, 1987.

Length of Treatment/Stay

Four to six weeks for cancer; one to three weeks for rheumatoid arthritis. Longer stays are available and sometimes recommended.

Costs

Treatment: $500 per day, including all lab fees, blood and urine analyses, and medicine.
Accommodations: $700 per week in the clinic.
Accompanying persons: $500 per week.

Method of Payment

Cash, money orders, and traveler's checks are accepted. Each week's payment must be made two weeks in advance.

Robert Janker Clinic

Fachklinik für Tumorerkrankungen
Baumschulallee 12–14
5300 Bonn 1
Germany

011–49–228–7291–0 (exchange)
011–49–228–7291–101 (secretary)
011–49–228–7291–164 (Mr. Simon)
Fax: 011–49–228–631832

Primary Personnel

Wolfgang Scheef, M.D., medical director.

Background

This is a 120-bed hospital near the center of the city.

Illness Treated

Cancer; the best responders are testicular, recurring breast, head and neck, all lymphomas, brain metastases, un-pretreated female genital, schwannoma, malignant oligodendroglioma, astrocytoma II–III, and medulloblastoma.

Treatment Offered

Integrated tumor therapy includes a special timing chemotherapy: a high concentration of it for a short time period in combination with radiation, hyperthermia, and immune stimulants such as water-soluble vitamin A emulsion, proteolytic enzymes, lipolytic enzymes, and other immune stimulants when appropriate.

Length of Treatment/Stay

Treatment consists of three therapy cycles. Each cycle lasts from 21 to 28 days after a rest of 15 to 20 days.

Costs

$150–$400* per day, depending on accommodations.

Method of Payment

Traveler's checks are accepted. Most insurance is accepted, but not Medicare.

Klinik Friedenweiler

Kurhausweg 2
D–7829 Friedenweiler 2
Germany

07651 208–0

Fax: 07651 208–116

Primary Personnel

Professor Dr. Albert Landsberger, medical superintendent.

Directions

On highway A5, the Frankfurt–Basel autoban, take the B31 turnoff to Freiburg in the direction of Titisee–Neustadt. After Neustadt, turn right to Friedenweiler.
By Train: Go to Neustadt and take a cab or make arrangements to be picked up.
By Plane: Go to Basel, from which Friedenweiler is one hour by land. It is one and a half hours from Stuttgart, two hours from Zurich, and three hours from Frankfurt.

*=Subject to the value of the U.S. dollar abroad.

Background

This clinic for biological cancer therapy and holistic medicine is situated in the Black Forest. Traditional European naturopathy and empirical medicine are combined with modern scientific medicine to address the physical, the personal, and the spiritual.

Illness Treated

Cancer and other diseases.

Treatment Offered

Chemical therapy with biological modification; mistletoe therapy; hormone therapy; thymus therapy; hydrotherapy; kinetotherapy; ergotherapy; psychotherapy; and biological therapy that includes induced fever treatments, ozone treatments, and tumor vaccinations. Dietary adaptation, pain treatment, and full diagnostic methods are part of the program, which also includes vitamins, minerals, enzymes, and trace elements.

Costs

Single room: $260* per day.
Double occupancy: $195* per day.

Method of Payment

Cash, cashier's checks, and traveler's checks are accepted. Prepayment is due 10 days prior to arrival. The balance of the bill is to be paid in cash or traveler's checks prior to departure.

Koda Clinic

2–228 Sakuragaoka
Yao-Shi
Osaka Prefecture 581
Japan

(0729) 22–5300

*=Subject to the value of the U.S. dollar abroad.

Primary Personnel

Mitsuo Koda, M.D.

Directions

Near Kintetsu Yao station, in the eastern part of Osaka Prefecture, between Osaka and Nara.

Background

Dr. Koda has spent 40 years conducting research into fasting and special diets (such as eating raw foods only) and using his expertise in that field to treat patients. His clinic has 20 beds and also offers outpatient treatment.

Illness Treated

Effective to some degree on all cancers; most responsive are cancers of the breast, lung, bladder, stomach, and large intestine.

Also effective for the auto-immune system and for treating arthritis, hepatitis, diabetes, and liver and kidney diseases.

Treatment Offered

Diet, fasting, exercise (Nishi style), cold and hot baths, information, support, and informal counseling.

Length of Treatment/Stay

Two weeks is the minimum stay, but many patients stay longer, some for six months.

Costs

Costs not submitted for publication.

Method of Payment

Japanese insurance is accepted. If your insurance company is based elsewhere, you will need to contact it to see what it covers.

Lukas Klinik

CH–4144 Arlesheim
Switzerland

(011) 41–61–72–3333

Directions

Take the tram from Basel. From Aeschenplatz to Arlesheim-Hirsland in 25 minutes. It's then a two-minute walk to the clinic.

Background

Lukas Klinik was founded in 1963 by R. & A. Leroi, who based Lukas on anthroposophical medicine. This 48-bed clinic is five miles south of Basel. The modern rooms have private bathrooms, some with baths as well. The clinic offers vegetarian meals, gardens, and lectures.

The staff of 12 physicians assesses progress daily. Laboratory and X-ray facilities are available. They treat mostly tumor diseases.

This clinic is regarded as one of the most completely holistic treatment centers in existence, addressing all aspects of the body, mind, and spirit.

Illness Treated

Cancer, especially in the early stages, of the breast, stomach, colon, rectum, bladder, ovaries, and lungs. The clinic treats all sorts of internal diseases.

Treatment Offered

Iscador—pressed juice of the Viscum album, a white-berried toxic mistletoe plant used in medicine for centuries—is injected. This particular treatment has been used since 1935 and is now used in many parts of Europe. Physical therapy—sauna, massage, medicinal baths. Artistic therapies—curative eurhythmics (movement), painting, modeling, speech formation, and color therapy. These artistic exercises were developed by Rudolf Steiner to heal all aspects of the being. Lectures and group discussions. The therapies have been used for 65 years.

Related Readings

"Misteltherapie, eine Antwort auf die Herausforderung Krebs. Die Pioniertat Rudolf Steiners und Ita Wegman" by Rita Leroi, 1987.

Over 200 additional publications by various authors.

Length of Treatment/Stay

Usually three to six weeks; four weeks is recommended.

Costs

Costs not submitted for publication.

Method of Payment

Cash only is accepted. No credit cards are accepted. Blue Cross covers hospital costs but not many of the adjunctive therapies.

Moerman Vereniging

Administratie
Postbus 14
6674 ZG Herveld
Netherlands

08880–1221

Contact Person

Doctors should contact Dr. Wagenaar, at Soestdijkerstraatweg 5, 1213 VP Hilversum, Netherlands, or by telephoning 035–210–000. Patients have a different contact and should telephone 08819–71579 or 08370–23950.

Background

Only two countries have Moerman doctors: Holland and Belgium. The doctors prevent and combat cancer by having the patient take certain vitamins and minerals and adopt a particular diet and lifestyle.

Members of Moerman Vereniging are cancer victims treated by the therapy of Dr. Moerman. Some people who sympathize but are not cancer victims have also joined.

Illness Treated

Cancer.

Treatment Offered

New patients call 08819–71579 or 08370–23950 to learn the name and phone number of that day's volunteer, who in turn will supply the address and phone number of a Moerman doctor who can accept the patient very soon for a short visit (about one hour). The volunteer will also supply the phone number of a person who has recovered from the same kind of cancer and the phone number of a nearby person who can accompany the patient to the doctor.

The patient receives a diet list, which the patient can start following even before visiting the doctor. The diet allows many foods (such as buttermilk, brown rice, cooked vegetables, pea soup, whole wheat bread, and almost all fruits), disallows many foods (such as meat, fish, poultry, coffee, tea, white-flour products, and yogurt), and makes lifestyle suggestions (such as no drinking of alcoholic beverages, no smoking, and avoiding sunbathing and other people's tobacco smoke).

The vitamins and minerals involved in the treatment are usually taken orally and require the doctor's prescription.

Related Readings

Dr. Moerman's Anti-Cancer Diet: Holland's Revolutionary Nutritional Program for Combatting Cancer by Ruth Jochems. Avery Publishing Group, 1990.

Length of Treatment/Stay

Patients stay at their own homes and see their Moerman doctor once a month.

Costs

The doctor and the chemist have to be paid. (All others involved are volunteers.) Their estimated fees were not submitted for publication.

Manuel D. Navarro, M.D.

3553 Sining Street
Morning Side Terrace
Santa Mesa, Manila 1008
Philippines

61–26–92
61–42–68

Office:
Room 108, UST Hospital
8–10 a.m.; 731–3001 Loc. (239)

Background

This program consists of early detection of cancer by an immuno-assay test of urine extract. Earliest detection has been 29 months prior to any symptoms.

There is an inpatient medical hospital with lab and X-ray facilities. For information on the test, contact Dr. Navarro at the above address or Mrs. Erlinda N. Suarez, 631 Peregrine Drive, Palatine, Illinois 60067, United States.

Illness Treated

Cancer.

Treatment Offered

Nontoxic metabolic therapy; vitamins B_{17}, A, B, C, E, K, and B_{15}; diet regimen; minerals; and immunotherapy.

Related Readings

A Program for Prevention and Detection of Pre-Cancerous Conditions by Walter Ermer, D.D. This is available from the Cancer Book House.

Vitamin B_{17}—Forbidden Weapon Against Cancer by Michael Culbert is also available from the Cancer Book House.

Costs

For a stay at the hospital, rooms are $10–$20* per day. Medication costs $10–$40* per day, depending on the dosage. Doctors' fees are $25–$60* per day, depending on the number of attending consultants.

*=Subject to the value of the U.S. dollar abroad.

Method of Payment

United States dollars and traveler's checks are accepted.

Hans A. Nieper, M.D.

Outpatient Office:
Sedan Strasse 21
3000 Hannover 1
Germany

011–49–511–348–08–08
Fax: 011–49–511–318417

Inpatient Clinic:
Paracelsus Klinik at Silbersee
Oertzeweg 24
3012 Langenhagen
Germany

011–49–511–7794–0
Fax: 011–49–511–778254

Contact Person

Nurse Monica; Mrs. Otte (office); Mrs. Koch (hospital).

Primary Personnel

Dr. Hans Nieper, director of department of medicine.

Directions

Hannover is north of Frankfurt.

Background

Dr. Nieper is the founder of the German Society of Medical Tumor Therapy, and he researched electrolyte carriers (mineral transporters), which led to the development of his eumetabolic therapy. In 1972, he founded a deshielding therapy as well. He was president of the German Society of Oncology from 1982 to 1985.

Outpatients see Dr. Nieper at his office. It is necessary to make reservations. Call from 9 a.m. to 4 p.m. (German time), preferably at 9 a.m. for an appointment. Confirm the appointment by letter. You can stay in a nearby hotel.

For the inpatient program, you will stay at the hospital in Silbersee. Call from noon to 4 p.m. (German time) for reservations. Confirm by letter. Guests or companions can stay in a nearby hotel or in a private room or guest house. Bring along a tape recorder.

For discount travel reservations (or for one of Dr. Nieper's books), contact Karen Dahl at Hansa Referral in the United States via telephone at (608) 637–3030 or via fax at (608) 637–7978.

Illness Treated

Cancer, multiple sclerosis, arteriosclerosis, coronary disease, amyotrophic lateral sclerosis, rheumatoid arthritis, and osteoporosis.

Treatment Offered

Eumetabolic therapy at early stages of cancer. Therapy includes direct treatment of tumors (one way is with gene repair); improvement and restoration of the body's defenses; immune status assessment; and overcoming the blocking and shielding phenomenon. Other therapeutic tools used are beta-carotene, laetrile, and zinc.

Related Readings

A list of all Dr. Nieper's publications can be obtained from Brewer Science Library, Richland Center, Wisconsin 53581, United States, telephone (608) 647–6513. Materials are in German, Spanish, French, and English. One of his books is *Dr. Nieper's Revolution in Technology, Medicine and Society.*

Length of Treatment/Stay

Depends on the health of the individual, but generally about 8–14 days. An appointment is required.

Costs

Outpatient therapy: approximately $1,500*, but check, as costs vary.
Inpatient therapy: 450–550 deutsche marks per day, which includes the doctor's fee and all treatment costs. May be more with severe illness. Deposit is required.

*=Subject to the value of the U.S. dollar abroad.

Method of Payment

All bills are to be paid in cash (deutsch marks) or United States traveler's checks (but only in deutsch marks). Private insurance has been reimbursing 75% on the average.

Nutrition & Stress Control Centre

One Trackson Street
Alderley 4051
Brisbane
Queensland
Australia

(07) 352–6634
Fax: (07) 356–5787

Contact Person

Nicole Wray; Helen Fowler.

Primary Personnel

Ruth Cilento, M.B., B.S., D.B.M., D.Ac., D.N.M.

Directions

At the corner of Enoggera Road and Trackson Street in Alderley. The centre is three kilometers (1.86 miles) from the Brisbane General Post Office. You may reach the centre by taxi or by Council Bus 172 (bus stop 24).

Background

Dr. Ruth Cilento graduated in medicine and surgery from Queensland University in 1949. After 20 years as a physician in general practice, she studied psychiatry and ran a government psychiatric outpatient clinic in a country hospital.

Dr. Cilento has run workshops and seminars on cancer and its treatments and has lectured on the subject, too. Since 1983, she has helped many patients in her private practice by teaching them orthomolecular stress control coupled with nutritional lessons. New patients undergo an all-day program, with lectures and tests, to teach them how to take the treatment prescribed. All treatments are on an outpatient basis only.

Illness Treated

Cancer. Also multiple sclerosis, arthritis, asthma, arteriosclerosis, Parkinson's disease, and other degenerative and immune system disorders.

Treatment Offered

Nutritional therapy depends on the disease and on an assessment of the individual, but it is based on fruit and vegetable juices; unadulterated, unprocessed foods; vitamins; minerals; gland extracts; protein derivatives; and enzymes to normalize the body's metabolic chemistry.

Other therapies used are herbal compounds, Hasumi autogenous vaccines, meditation and visual imagery, relaxation techniques, group support, and home nursing information. If appropriate, Gerson therapy may be used.

Emphasis is on teaching the patient and family to take responsibility for administering the treatments at home. Follow-up consultations are recommended every eight weeks.

Related Readings

In Search of Cancer Answers by Dr. Ruth Cilento.

Getting Well Again by O. Carl Simonton, Stephanie Matthews-Simonton, and James Creighton.

You Can Conquer Cancer by Ian Gawler.

Anatomy of an Illness by Norman Cousins.

Where There's Hope by Patricia Gilshennan.

Cancer and its Nutritional Therapies by Richard Passwater and others.

Access to a network of recovered past patients is permitted in select instances.

Length of Treatment/Stay

Initial contact varies from one day to two weeks, depending on the availability of test results. To establish a stable recovery, follow-up could occur at intervals of two to three months and continue for a period of three to five years.

Costs

First consultation: $100.
Full-day seminar: $350.
Follow-up consultation: $65–$70.
Quality-of-life support group meetings: Free. (Held each Friday.)
A Medicare rebate of $50 is applicable. Family members may attend any of the above for a reduced fee. Patients will need to arrange for accommodations in any of the Brisbane motels.

Method of Payment

Australian dollars and Australian bank drafts are accepted. All fees must be paid in advance. Private insurance companies generally pay 85% of each cost but will not pay for the seminar.

Park Attwood Clinic

Trimpley, Bewdley
Worcestershire
DY12 1RE
England
United Kingdom

02997–444
Fax: 02997–375

Contact Person

Stephen Moore, administrator.

Primary Personnel

Dr. Maurice Orange; Dr. Frank A. Mulder.

Background

Park Attwood is registered under the English nursing home and residential home system for 13 and 11 beds, respectively. It has a maximum capacity of 20 beds. The two doctors are supported by a team of ten registered nurses, three artistic therapists, and two masseurs. The doctors prescribe mainly anthroposophical (homeopathy-based) medicines but will prescribe allopathic medicines where appropriate.

Illness Treated

Cancer in its many forms, rheumatic conditions, nervous system afflictions (particularly multiple sclerosis), and all forms of anxiety-related conditions (from life crises to mild forms of psychosis).

Treatment Offered

The regime at Park Attwood begins with consultations with the doctors, who, in addition to prescribing medicines, are able to choose artistic therapy (painting, sculpture, and movement), rhythmical or hauschke massage, and speech therapy. Diet and the social life in the house provide support to the overall treatment.

Related Readings

Extending the Art of Healing by Dr. Michael R. Evans.

Anthroposophical Medicine by Victor Bott, M.D.

Anthroposophically Orientated Medicine and its Remedies by Otto Wolff. Mercury Press, Spring Valley.

Length of Treatment/Stay

Varies dramatically, but the average stay is 3–6 weeks.

Costs

Park Attwood operates on a policy of admission by medical need. Health insurance companies pay 120 pounds per day for patients with policies who stay at Park Attwood. Otherwise, financial arrangements are made by individual negotiation.

Method of Payment

Payment in any form should be received within 30 days of date of discharge. Checks drawn on banks from outside the United Kingdom are acceptable but will result in a 1% fee to cover bank charges.

Veramed Klinik am Wendelstein

D–8204 Brannenburg/Obb.
Germany

08034/3020
Fax: 08034/7835

Contact Person

Mr. Schuster (telephone 08034/302750).

Primary Personnel

Peter Holzhauer, M.D., and Georg Frank, M.D., medical directors.

Directions

This clinic is 45 minutes south of Munich. It is in the mountains on the road to Innsbruck, which is 50 minutes away.

Background

This hospital synthesizes traditional and alternative therapeutic approaches. The cancer program is designed to strengthen the immune system as well as repair damage from the stresses of surgery, radiation, and chemotherapy. There is an intensive care unit within the clinic.

Illness Treated

Cancer and other chronic degenerative diseases.

Treatment Offered

Chemotherapy, hormone therapy, local perfusion therapy, oxygen and ozone therapies, immune therapy (using interferon, interleukens, TNF, and thymus), fever therapy, hyperthermia, pain therapy, nutritional guidance and supervision, psychological therapies, diagnostic services, medical massages (including connective tissue), Fango, medicinal baths, lymphatic drainage, colon therapy, magnetic therapies, microwave, and diathermy.

Length of Treatment/Stay

Approximately 30 days.

Costs

Semiprivate room for inpatients: $260* per day.
Private room for inpatients: $300* per day.
Total cost: approximately $450* per day.

*=Subject to the value of the U.S. dollar abroad.

Method of Payment

Cash, cashier's checks, and traveler's checks are accepted. A $10,000* deposit is required in advance. For insurance purposes, three itemized bills are presented: one for room and board, one for medication, and one for medical services.

Wessex Cancer Help Centre

8 South Street
Chichester
West Sussex PO19 1EH
England
United Kingdom

(0243) 778516

Contact Person

David Holmes, chairman; Betty Deal, coordinator.

Primary Personnel

David Holmes, F.R.S.H., M.I.H.E., F.S.A.E., F.R.S.A., Dip.Ed.

Directions

The centre is in the south of England, approximately 90 minutes from London.

Background

The centre was founded in 1982 to treat cancer sufferers holistically. It follows the philosophy of the Bristol Cancer Help Centre. Two-thirds of its work concentrates on prevention. Its large team of doctors, practitioners, counselors, and ministers works to provide treatment and support for patients and their families. The centre does not have residential facilities.

*=Subject to the value of the U.S. dollar abroad.

Illness Treated

Mainly cancer, but the centre will deal with all degenerative illnesses.

Treatment Offered

Diets, acupuncture, psychotherapy, counseling, relaxation, biofeedback, homeopathy, hypno-therapy, visualization, vitamin therapy, and mineral therapy.

Related Readings

New Hope and Improved Treatments for Cancer Patients by David Holmes.

Recipe Book by Wessex Cancer Help Centre.

New Approaches to Cancer by Shirley Harrison. Century.

Fight Cancer by Professor Karol Sikora and Dr. Hilary Thomas. BBC Books.

Bristol Detox Diet by Dr. Alec Forbes. Keats/Pivot.

Cancer and its Nutritional Therapies by Richard A. Passwater. Keats/Pivot.

Costs

The centre is a charity. Most of its information, including all of its preventative advice, is offered for free. To cover the costs of printing, the centre's package of literature carries a price of 2.5 pounds. Doctors and practitioners will charge each patient for any services they perform. Doctors' costs not submitted for publication.

Educational Centers

Institutes, Organizations, Physicians, Health Practitioners

North America (United States)

Biological Immunity Research Institute

6821 East Thomas Road
Scottsdale, Arizona 85251
United States

(602) 945–3876
(800) 654–3734

Contact Person

Geneva or Donna.

Primary Personnel

Gary A. Martin, D.Sc., Ph.D.

Directions

Located in Scottsdale, Arizona, a suburb on the east side of Phoenix.

Background

The institute analyzes biological immunity by examining urine and saliva. The analysis indicates what may be causing the illness so a complete program can be prepared to restore the immune system.

Illness Addressed

The institute accepts all chronic degenerative cases.

Type of Program Offered

Diet, nutrition, lifestyle changes, and stress management. After first sending specific information regarding the particular illness, the client should call the office to make an appointment. At the same time, the patient should ask the staff to make arrangements at a nearby motel if needed. Consultations usually start at 8:30 a.m. each day. The institute recommends that the client send for initial paperwork and specimen kit and complete the necessary forms.

Related Readings

The Biological Immunity Analysis by Gary A. Martin, D.Sc., Ph.D., 1990.

Nutripathy—The Final Solution to Your Health Dilemma by Gary A. Martin, D.Sc., Ph.D., 1976.

Don't Eat the Yellow Snow by Gary A. Martin, D.Sc., Ph.D., 1987.

Length of Program/Stay

Two weeks for acute problems; four weeks for chronic disorders. It is also possible to complete the program by remaining home and working with the institute by sending specimens via overnight mail.

Costs

Motel: $250 per week.
Two-week treatment: $1,990. Includes lab fees, urinalysis, physical, counseling, and therapies.
Four-week treatment: $3,990.
Additional items such as enzymes, amino acids, and other supplements are extra.
By mail, the analysis is $195 for the first month and $90 for each successive month.

Method of Payment

Full payment is made on the first day. Personal checks are accepted. Papers will be completed for possible reimbursement from your insurance company.

Creative Health Institute

918 Union City Road
Union City, Michigan 49094
United States

(517) 278–6260

Directions

Union City is south of Battle Creek. Take Coldwater Road east out of Union City. It becomes Union City Road heading southeast. The institute is in Hodunk.

Background

Creative Health Institute is directly affiliated with Dr. Ann Wigmore. The institute teaches a "living foods" lifestyle and offers people an opportunity to learn in a hands-on program. The ultimate goal of the center is to help people help themselves in body, mind, and spirit. The center is situated on 300 acres along the banks of a river. This particular center has been open for 11 years and can accommodate 25 people.

Illness Addressed

The center welcomes people who are able to care for themselves. If people are unable to do this, they may bring someone to tend to their physical needs. Guests and companions pay the regular program price. The center is not in a position to accept AIDS patients as guests.

Type of Program Offered

The program consists of courses and lectures on different aspects of health and cleansing; there are daily exercise classes, meditation and relaxation periods, etc. A large part of the institute's focus is the hands-on experimental learning process addressing things such as sprouting, growing greens indoors, living food preparation, etc.

Related Readings

Be Your Own Doctor: A Positive Guide to Natural Living by Ann Wigmore. Avery Publishing Group, 1982.

Recipes for a Longer Life by Ann Wigmore. Avery Publishing Group, 1978.

The Sprouting Book by Ann Wigmore. Avery Publishing Group, 1986.

The Wheatgrass Book by Ann Wigmore. Avery Publishing Group, 1985.

Why Suffer? by Ann Wigmore. Avery Publishing Group, 1985.

The center also has a list of mail-order books.

Length of Program/Stay

The typical program length is two weeks. Discounts are available for longer stays.

Costs

Standard cost: $390 per week.
Semiprivate: $460 per week.
Private: $580 per week.
All costs include classes, meals, and room.

Method of Payment

Cash, checks, and money orders are accepted.

Health Action

19 East Mission Street, Suite 102
Santa Barbara, California 93101
United States

(805) 682–3230

Contact Person

Gael Ashwood.

Primary Personnel

Roger Jahnke, doctor of oriental medicine (O.M.D.).

Directions

Take West Coast Highway 101. Santa Barbara is 100 miles north of Los Angeles, 350 miles south of San Francisco. Take Mission Street exit.

Background

The underlying concept is that energy in the body must flow freely or disease ensues. Health Action assists in activating the body's self-healing mechanisms, resulting in physiological and emotional balance.

Illness Addressed

Acute/chronic pain, anxiety, depression, insomnia, low energy, fatigue, immune deficiency, digestive dysfunction, all the symptoms that accompany cancer, and the side effects of chemotherapy and radiological therapy.

Type of Program Offered

Acupuncture, herbal medicine, nutrition, stress management, therapeutic massage, hypnotherapy, physical therapy, and self-care guidance (biofeedback, relaxation techniques, self-esteem, and visualization).

Related Readings

The Self-Applied Health Enhancement Methods by Roger Jahnke, O.M.D., published by Health Action.

The Most Profound Medicine by Roger Jahnke, O.M.D., published by Health Action.

The Web That Has No Wearer by Ted Kaptchuk, O.M.D.

The Relaxation Response by Herbert Benson, M.D.

Encounters With Qi by Dr. Eisenburg.

Length of Program/Stay

Varies with each patient.

Costs

$80 for an initial consultation.
$65 per treatment (10% discount for immediate payment).

Method of Payment

Personal checks, cash, MasterCard, and Visa are accepted. Insurance is accepted, but check with insurance company first for coverage of acupuncture and physical therapy.

Hippocrates Health Institute

1443 Palmdale Court
West Palm Beach, Florida 33411
United States

(407) 471–8876
(800) 842–2125

Contact Person

Ask for program counselors or for reservations.

Primary Personnel

Brian and Anna Marie Clement, directors.

Directions

Take Florida turnpike to Okeechobee exit (West Palm Beach). Turn right onto Okeechobee Road to first light (Skees Road). Turn left onto Skees and go three quarters of a mile to Palmdale Road. Turn right; then take first right onto Palmdale Court. Go to the end of the street. The institute is ten minutes from West Palm Beach International Airport.

Background

For more than 35 years, Hippocrates Health has pioneered the development of a lifestyle program of nutrition through living foods, moderate exercise, and stress reduction. The concept of living foods began in the United States more than four decades ago with Hippocrates founder Ann Wigmore and a dedicated group of health pioneers.

Through extensive research and experimentation, Hippocrates Health has continued to update its health restoration program, and today it enjoys a worldwide reputation among professionals and lay people. Its program consists of a cleansing and nourishing diet of raw foods integrated with a range of holistic therapies. The program teaches a plan of gradual transition to a more healthful lifestyle that people can implement in their daily lives.

Illness Addressed

All types of cancer and degenerative diseases.

Type of Program Offered

The program includes a special diet consisting of uncooked vegetables, fresh fruits, sprouted seeds, grains, and beans. Wheatgrass juice therapy is usually prescribed. There are daily classes in exercise, human physiology, body purification, detoxification, food preparation, sprouting, and stress management. Also available are massages, electromagnetic treatments, an oxygenated pool, and a sauna. Plus the services of its professional non-residential staff: medical doctor, dentist, colon therapist, chiropractor, psychologist, psychoneuro-immunology specialist, and aesthetician.

Related Readings

Be Your Own Doctor: A Positive Guide to Natural Living by Ann Wigmore. Avery Publishing Group, 1982.

Belief by Brian Clement. Hippocrates Publications, 1991.

The Hippocrates Diet and Health Program by Ann Wigmore. Avery Publishing Group, 1984.

How I Conquered Cancer Naturally by Eydie Mae Hunsberger. Harvest House, 1985.

The Wheatgrass Book by Ann Wigmore. Avery Publishing Group, 1985.

Hippocrates Health Program: A Proven Guide to Healthful Living by Brian Clement. Hippocrates Publications, 1990.

(The center will in some cases provide information regarding past patients.)

Length of Program/Stay

Three weeks recommended. Stays of one or two weeks are also available.

Costs

On-site accommodations range from $125 per day for a dormitory room to $300 per day for a private deluxe room. Costs include all meals, classes, activities, one massage per week, electro-magnetic treatments, private consultations with the directors, live cell analysis, and clinical bloodwork.

Some people may want to join the program but live off premises. Hippocrates Health will admit up to 12 such students into its program. Each non-resident student pays $2,000 for three weeks. Plus, for those with a trailer or mobile home, the Pine Lake Camp Resort for recreational vehicles is only minutes away.

Method of Payment

Money orders, cashier's checks, American Express, MasterCard, and Visa are accepted. Some insurance is accepted. To secure a place in the program, students must make reservations, either over the telephone by using one of the accepted credit cards or by mailing a non-refundable deposit of half the total cost. Any balance due is payable upon arrival at the institute.

International Association for Oxygen Therapy

P.O. Box 1360
Priest River, Idaho 83856
United States

(208) 448–2504

Contact Person

Arlene Steiner, R.N.C., B.S.

Primary Personnel

G.A. Freibott, N.D., M.D.

Background

A division of the American Society of Medical Missionaries, the International Oxidation Institute was reorganized and renamed the International Association for Oxygen Therapy in 1983. The organization's primary focus is the training and placement of "oxidation therapists" and medical missionaries. It offers many acres of retreat space. A center with expanded training/classes on oxidation and on the interaction of all bodily diseases is under construction. It will have space to accommodate ten people as an inpatient facility with organic, simple, and God-related beliefs.

Illness Addressed

This organization does not treat illnesses, but it helps teach the restoration of proper oxidation/oxidative body and natural functioning based on the teachings of Fr. Kneipp; Otto Warburg; F.M. Eugene Blass; Dr. W.F. Koch; and the scriptures.

Type of Program Offered

Classes involve the following: 1. Hydrotherapy: colonics, hot tub, and sauna. 2. Education in sprouting, wheatgrass, diet alterations, cooking, and uncooking. 3. Naturopathy, homeopathy, Koch therapy, Blass' oxygen therapy, Ipe Roxo teas, and Mucorhicin. 4. Bible study.

Related Readings

Contact the association for any information regarding related classes and historical data.

Length of Program/Stay

Two weeks to twelve months, depending on need and commitment. This is lifestyle training, not a treatment per se.

Costs

Individually determined. It can range from $100 to $2,000 biweekly in donations.

Method of Payment

Work trades and some apprentice positions may be open. Financial support is a must and is appreciated.

Kushi Institute

P.O. Box 7
Becket, Massachusetts 01223
United States

(413) 623–5741

Primary Personnel

Michio Kushi.

Background

The Kushi Institute (a division of the Kushi Foundation) is directed by educators Michio and Aveline Kushi. The Kushi Institute teaches the macrobiotic approach to health, happiness, and peace. Courses are offered in macrobiotic cooking, Far Eastern and traditional Western philosophy, macrobiotic medicine, modern nutrition, Shiatsu massage, family and community harmony, and world peace. There are also ongoing lectures, seminars, and programs of shorter duration.

During the past 15 years, the Kushis and their associates have developed a comprehensive approach to preventing and treating degenerative diseases, especially cancer, heart disease, and AIDS. Research studies at Harvard Medical School, the Framingham Heart Study, Boston University, and elsewhere have begun to determine the value of the macrobiotic approach. The Kushi Institute's emphasis is on each person and each family taking responsibility for their own health and happiness.

The Kushi Foundation and the Kushi Institute are not medical clinics, nor do they offer medical diagnosis or treatment. They offer public education to persons interested in learning more about this traditional way of life.

The Kushi Institute also has several locations in Europe.

Illness Addressed

Cancer, degenerative diseases, and AIDS.

Type of Program Offered

The Kushi Foundation offers a two-day program entitled *The Macrobiotic Way of Life Seminar*, Parts 1 and 2, which provides basic (Part 1) and more advanced (Part 2) information on the macrobiotic way of life, including lectures, demonstrations, cooking classes, and, if requested, a private interview in practicing the proper way of life to improve health and well-being.

The Kushi Foundation also offers a seven-day residential program in a warm and cozy group setting, with classes, lectures, and demonstrations on the basics of macrobiotic living. It also offers a four-day spiritual development program, which consists of 12 levels.

Related Readings

The Cancer-Prevention Diet by Michio Kushi and Alex Jack. St. Martin's Press, 1985.

The Macrobiotic Approach to Cancer by Michio Kushi with Ed Esko. Second edition. Avery Publishing Group, 1991.

The Macrobiotic Cancer Prevention Cookbook by Aveline Kushi with Wendy Esko. Avery Publishing Group, 1988.

Macrobiotic Diet by Michio Kushi with Alex Jack. Tokyo: Japan Publications, 1985.

The Macrobiotic Way by Michio Kushi and Steven Blauer. Avery Publishing Group, 1985.

The Changing Seasons Macrobiotic Cookbook by Aveline Kushi and Wendy Esko. Avery Publishing Group, 1985.

These books and others, plus video and audio tapes, macrobiotic foods, and cookware, are available by mail order through the foundation.

Length of Program/Stay

There are three levels of study, each level lasting five weeks.

Costs

Macrobiotic way of life seminar: $250; $175 for an accompanying support person. Seven-day residential program (including room and board): $895; $695 for an accompanying support person. Four-day spiritual development program: $495 for each level of development; $895 for two levels if taken back-to-back.

Method of Payment

Visa, MasterCard, American Express, checks, and money orders are accepted as payment through the mail.

If you do not live near the Kushi Institute but are interested in learning more about macrobiotics in the United States, you may wish to contact one of the following educational centers. While these centers are not necessarily associated with the Kushi Institute, in many cases they will be able to provide you with information and/or training regarding the macrobiotic lifestyle.

Catskill Macrobiotic Center
100 Washington Avenue
Saugerties, New York 12477

(914) 246–4168

East West Center for Macrobiotics
1122 M Street
Eureka, California 95501

(707) 445–2290

Health Education Action Liaison
Department of Residential Programs
835 7th Street
Santa Monica, California 90403

(213) 395–6938

Health Education Action Liaison
Department of Education and Research
144 West 16th Street, No. 9
New York, New York 10011

(212) 243–6051

Kushi Macrobiotic Center of Northern New Jersey
33 Market Street
Morristown, New Jersey 07960

(201) 984–1616

Los Angeles East West Center
11215 Hannum Avenue
Culver City, California 90230

(213) 398–2228

Macrobiotic Association of Pennsylvania
606 South Ninth Street
Philadelphia, Pennsylvania 19147
(215) 483–9800

Macrobiotic Center of Dallas
14369 Haymeadow Circle
Dallas, Texas 75240
(214) 233–4938

Macrobiotic Center of Westchester, New York
89 Marble Avenue
Pleasantville, New York 10570
(914) 769–5083

Macrobiotic Education Center
15231 Kercheval Avenue, #5
Grosse Pointe Park, Michigan 48230
(313) 331–6900

Macrobiotic Foundation of Florida
3291 Franklin Avenue
Coconut Grove (Miami), Florida 33133
(305) 448–6625

Macrobiotic Grocery and Learning Center
1050 40th Street
Oakland, California 94608
(415) 653–6510

Northshore Macrobiotic Center
P.O. Box 1122
Gloucester, Massachusetts 01930
(617) 738–0045

Vega Macrobiotic Center
1511 Robinson Street
Oroville, California 95965
(916) 533–7702

Optimum Health Institute of San Diego

6970 Central Avenue
Lemon Grove, California 91945
United States

(619) 464–3346
Fax: (619) 589–4098

Primary Personnel

Robert P. Nees, director; Raychel Solomon, founder.

Background

This is a premiere holistic health center. The program is based on a 100% living foods diet to eliminate body toxins. There is an open house every Sunday at 4:30 p.m., if you want to visit. The facility has a maximum capacity of 125 guests. The program itself starts on Sundays. Dress casually, and bring a swimsuit for the whirlpool bath.

Illness Addressed

Illnesses are not addressed. Emphasis is on wellness.

Type of Program Offered

Diet and exercise. The living foods diet includes: sprouts, greens, fruits, vegetables, enzymatic seed sauces, juices, enzyme-rich rejuvelac, sauerkraut, and wheatgrass juice. The facility also provides classes dealing with exercise, nutrition, positive thinking, and emotional and spiritual support.

Related Readings

Survival into the 21st Century by Viktoras Kulvinskas. Omangod Press, 1975.

Coming Alive with Raychel by Raychel Solomon and Dr. Mark Solomon.

Books, cassette tapes, and equipment to maintain lifestyle as it is taught in this program are available through mail order.

Length of Program/Stay

Three-week stays are recommended, but shorter stays are accepted.

Costs

A $50 deposit per week of stay is required two weeks before arrival.
Private room: $365 per week.
Double room: $265 per week per person.
Two-bedroom townhouse: $450 per week if just one person; $365 per person per week if two people.
Executive suite: $500 per person/$850 per couple each week.
This fee includes room, meals, linens, lectures, and classes, and is to be paid in full upon arrival. At extra cost are books and equipment.

Method of Payment

Traveler's checks, money orders, cashier's checks, MasterCard, Visa, personal checks, and cash are accepted.

Linus Pauling Institute of Science and Medicine

440 Page Mill Road
Palo Alto, California 94306
United States

(415) 327–4064
Fax: (415) 327–8564

Primary Personnel

Dr. Linus Pauling; Richard Hicks.

Background

The institute works primarily at researching vitamin C applications to orthomolecular and preventive approaches to medicine. Dr. Pauling is a two-time Nobel Laureate.

Illness Addressed

Research areas include cancer, AIDS, cardiovascular disease, and aging.

Type of Program Offered

The institute's recommended dosage of vitamin C is specific. This dosage is said by the institute to be helpful to virtually every cancer patient; the effects can be quite dramatic for a fortunate few.

The general recommendation on how to proceed with taking vitamin C each day is described in literature from the institute. It is important that vitamin C therapy be consistent and be maintained indefinitely, once the dose is decided upon. If there should be any need to discontinue the therapy, decrease the dosage gradually.

Vitamin C has remarkably low toxicity and few side effects.

Note: Patients who have been placed on low-salt diets by their physicians should not use sodium ascorbate (vitamin C). Ten grams of sodium ascorbate equal approximately three grams of sodium chloride (table salt).

Information on AIDS treatments is also available.

Related Readings

Cancer and Vitamin C by Ewan Cameron and Linus Pauling. Linus Pauling Institute of Science and Medicine, 1979.

How to Live Longer and Feel Better by Linus Pauling. 1986.

Costs

Tax deductible donations.

Project Cure

1101 Connecticut Avenue N.W.
Washington, DC 20036
United States

5910 North Central Expressway
Suite 760
Dallas, Texas 75206
United States

(214) 891–6111
Fax: (214) 891–6115

Primary Personnel

Michael S. Evers, J.D., president; Sheri Patrick, executive secretary.

Background

Established in 1979 as a pro-consumer lobby by Robert DeBragga, a recovering cancer patient, Project Cure has become a leading force in the continuing struggle to have alternative therapies objectively investigated and accepted by mainstream medicine. The non-profit organization lobbies Congress to provide funding for alternative therapy research and to ensure a more balanced debate on all health issues in which consumers have a stake, such as access to services, quality of care, cost containment, and freedom of choice between different practitioners and services.

Mr. Evers, an attorney with extensive experience in alternative medico-legal issues, was commissioned by the congressional Office of Technology Assessment (OTA) to prepare an exhaustive report on the legal constraints faced by those who employ or seek to use alternative cancer treatments in the United States. OTA's final report, issued in September 1990, confirmed that although several alternative therapies show promise of benefit, the National Cancer Institute has failed to investigate them objectively and continues to ignore important evidence of potentially useful nutritional and nontoxic treatments.

Project Cure finances political and historical medical research, sponsors educational conferences and policy forums, and distributes special reports to Congress, the media, and the public. Project Cure's mission is to have nutritional and other nontoxic cancer therapies available to medical practitioners and their patients as a part of standard medical practice. It believes that informed patients, not the government or the medical establishment, should have the final say regarding what therapies they may employ to treat themselves and their families.

Illness Addressed

Cancer and related life-threatening diseases.

Type of Program Offered

Mail-order books, articles, videos, special reports, and newsletters are available, many free of charge. In addition, Project Cure maintains a clearinghouse for information about alternative medico-legal issues.

Costs

Contributions of any amount are accepted to further Project Cure's work. Since it is a lobbying organization and not a charity, contributions are not tax deductible.

Method of Payment

Checks, Visa, MasterCard, and money orders are accepted.

Southeast Research Foundation Inc.

5416 Glen Cove Drive
Knoxville, Tennessee 37919
United States

(615) 588–7678
(615) 584–8150

Contact Person

Chris Poole, treasurer.

Background

The foundation was founded in 1983 by Dr. Cecil Pitard, who was stricken with cancer in 1981 and given a prognosis of six months to live. He developed a protocol for the treatment of cancer and applied it to himself, adding another ten years to his life.

Illness Addressed

All types of cancer; good responses with leukemia, bone cancer, and brain tumors; but any other cancer—including breast cancer—can respond well, too, depending upon an individual's biochemistry and state of health.

Type of Program Offered

The foundation identifies and explains the use of Dr. Pitard's protocol of all-natural drugs and vitamins, some taken orally and others by injection. Information is offered to patients, doctors, and other interested parties. The foundation does not dispense the drugs, some of which require a physician's prescription. In all cases, a doctor's supervision is recommended. The patient will likely know within a month of being on the full program (taking all drugs prescribed) whether it will help or not.

Costs

The foundation is a non-profit organization and does not charge any fees. However, donations are welcome. Patients can purchase ingredients for the protocol for less than $3 per day of treatment.

Syracuse Cancer Research Institute Inc.

Presidential Plaza
600 East Genesee Street
Syracuse, New York 13202
United States

(315) 472–6616

Primary Personnel

Joseph Gold, M.D.

Background

Founded by its director, Dr. Joseph Gold, the institute began operations at its present location early in 1966. At the time, the cause of cancer cachexia—the weight loss and debilitation seen in cancer patients—was unknown. Dr. Gold found that the condition is largely the result of cancer's ability to "recycle wastes" at the energy expense of the body, thus imposing a severe energy drain on the body, eventually resulting in cachexia. Specifically, it was pointed out that cancer uses glucose (sugar) as its fuel but metabolizes it only incompletely.

Hydrazine sulfate is one of a new class of gluconeogenic blocking agents that functions as a specific chemotherapeutic agent for cancer cachexia. The drug, developed by the Syracuse Cancer Research Institute, has been in limited clinical use since late 1973. This substance, based on the work of Dr. Gold, is widely used in Russia; some of the clinics listed in this resource guide also use this chemical. Once considered an unproven method by the American Cancer Society, it now has the support of the American Cancer Society and the National Cancer Institute.

Illness Addressed

Cancer.

Type of Program Offered

Your doctor can write to the institute and receive an information packet for physicians; it includes reports on tests with hydrazine sulfate.

Related Readings

"Proposed Treatment of Cancer by Inhibition of Gluconeogenesis" by Joseph Gold, M.D. *Oncology* 22, pages 185–207, 1968.

Use of Hydrazine Sulfate in Terminal and Preterminal Cancer Patients: Preliminary Results (abstr.) by Joseph Gold, M.D., Proc Am Assoc Cancer Res 15, 83, 1974.

Additional articles and references are available to doctors from the institute.

Costs

Contributions to the cash fund are accepted. Contributions of equities are placed in the cash fund or in the endowment fund, depending on the donor's wishes. All contributions are tax deductible.

Method of Payment

Checks and money orders are accepted.

Ann Wigmore Foundation

196 Commonwealth Avenue
Boston, Massachusetts 02116
United States

(617) 267–9424

Ann Wigmore Research and Education Institute
Ruta 115, Km. 20
Barrio Guayabo
Aguada, Puerto Rico 00743
United States

Mailing Address:
P.O. Box 429
Ricon, Puerto Rico 00743

(809) 868–6307

Directions

Ann Wigmore Foundation in Boston—from highway I-95 take Massachusetts Avenue and turn right onto Commonwealth Avenue to 196. Ann Wigmore Research and Education Institute in Puerto Rico—fly into San Juan. A small commuter plane must then be taken to the western side of the island.

Background

Complete back-to-nature approach for overcoming all forms of disease. The use of high-enzyme easy-to-digest nourishment has been shown to help the body overcome illness and disease, including cancer. The theory that deficiency and toxemia are the two causes for all disease is taught.

Illness Addressed

All forms of illness. Patients who are not ambulatory are encouraged to go to the Puerto Rico center. If the condition is critical, first contact Dr. Ann to see if the patient can be accepted.

Type of Program Offered

A change in lifestyle. Many blended high-energy foods are used to replace deficiencies and remove toxins. Colon care, enemas, colonics, relaxation, wheatgrass therapy, mental and emotional balancing, and more. Emphasis is placed on self-sufficiency through the learn-by-doing program.

Related Readings

The Hippocrates Diet and Health Program by Ann Wigmore. Avery Publishing Group, 1984.

The Wheatgrass Book by Ann Wigmore. Avery Publishing Group, 1985.

Length of Program/Stay

Two-week program. In Boston, begins every other Monday and ends on a Saturday; in Puerto Rico, begins and ends in midweek. Longer stays can easily be arranged.

Costs

Dormitory room: $895.
Private room: $1,300.
These costs include all room and board, classes, instruction, private consultation with Dr. Ann, etc.

Method of Payment

Patients pay in full the first day. Personal checks, money orders, traveler's checks, and cash are accepted. No credit cards are taken at the Boston center.

Educational Centers

Institutes, Organizations, Physicians, Health Practitioners
Overseas (Australia, Japan, New Zealand, United Kingdom)

I.J. Bullen

297 Pearson Street
Woodlands
Western Australia 6018
Australia

09–4451994

Contact Person

Gail Lyon.

Primary Personnel

I.J. Bullen, MBBS, D.Obst. RCOG.

Directions

Take Mitchell Freeway northbound, exit at Powis Street, go straight ahead to Jon Sanders Drive. After passing through an industrial area, Jon Sanders Drive changes name to Pearson Street. The doctor's office is on the right, three houses before the Leige Street traffic lights. (Because of a median strip, you will need to go past the lights, turn around, and come back again.)

Background

Dr. Bullen is a general practitioner with an interest in the supportive care of cancer patients through meditation, counseling, nutrition, and three-day health retreats. Dr. Bullen is a member of the Australian College of Nutritional Medicine.

Type of Program Offered

General medical care, nutritional advice, intravenous vitamin C, counseling, meditation, allergy assessment, and three-day health retreats.

The retreats are held in fully equipped log cabins in a beautiful bushland setting in Jarrahdale Hills (about 45 minutes away). Each retreat commences Thursday night and concludes late Sunday afternoon. It is an intensive, positive, motivational, mind-training program. All meals are vegetarian, low in fat, and as close to 100% organic as the staff can manage. The retreats feature speakers on nutrition, therapeutic massage, Reiki, and other complementary therapies. To balance the holistic program, an oncologist and a radiotherapist speak about their specialties and about the structure and function of the immune system. In an informal, relaxed setting, patients pose questions and receive answers.

Related Readings

Man the Healer by Jose Silva.

Cancer and Vitamin C by Linus Pauling and Ewan Cameron.

Anatomy of an Illness by Norman Cousins.

You Can Knock Out AIDS With Vitamin C by Dr. Ian Brighthope.

Vitamin C as a Fundamental Medicine by Dr. London H. Smith.

Fight Fatigue by Dr. Ian Brighthope.

You Can Conquer Cancer by Ian Gawler.

Love, Medicine, and Miracles by Dr. Bernie Siegel.

Love, Peace, and Healing by Dr. Bernie Siegel.

Getting Well Again by O. Carl Simonton, Stephanie Matthews-Simonton, and James Creighton. J.P. Tarcher, 1978.

You Can Heal Your Life by Louise Hay.

Costs

Initial consultation (which is usually long): $80.
Ten-day course: $240 for vitamin C, plus a $30 consulting fee.
Follow-up vitamin C treatment: $23.50 per week for a 30 gram dose, plus a $30 consulting fee.
Cost of weekend retreat and other services not submitted for publication.
(All costs given in Australian dollars.)

Gawler Foundation Inc.

Yarra Valley Living Centre
P.O. Box 77G
Yarra Junction, 3797
Australia

(059) 67 1730

Contact Person

Diane Packer.

Primary Personnel

Dr. Ian Gawler, O.A.M., B.V. Sc., and Gayle Gawler, directors; Bob Sharples.

Background

All programs are based on the experiences of Ian and Gayle Gawler during Ian's recovery from a supposedly terminal bone cancer in 1975. They have worked with more than 5,000 patients since the programs began in 1981. They built on the results of that work and started the Gawler Foundation, which is a non-profit, nondenominational association of cancer patients, their families, and concerned individuals. Its goals are: to provide active support for cancer patients and their families, with the aim of improving quality and quantity of life; to give recognition to the importance of the patient's contribution to the outcome of the treatment; to encourage patients to play an active, positive role in getting well again; to focus on the significance of nutrition, stress, positive thinking, meditation, and self-help groups; to foster research into the significance of the patient's role in cancer; to provide access to educational facilities and to sponsor relevant lectures, seminars, and workshops; to facilitate access to ancillary services such as dietitians, counselors, masseurs, etc., as an adjunct to medical treatments; to encourage communication and cooperation between patients and medical personnel; to provide assistance to disadvantaged patients where appropriate; to encourage and sponsor the establishment of affiliated self-help groups; and to take an active role in disseminating to the public information regarding cancer prevention.

Illness Addressed

Cancer.

Type of Program Offered

A 12-week support group designed for cancer patients, their families, and their friends. The group meets for two hours each week.

In Yarra Valley, there is a five-day residential program that creates an opportunity to review your life situation, seek clarity about your future direction, find meaning and purpose in your life, learn and practice self-help techniques, and experience meditation.

Costs

Support group: $150 (Australian) per series of 12 weekly sessions; $90 (Australian) for extra people.
Yarra Valley: $675 (Australian) for full residential program at Jumbunna Lodge.

Herbal Education Resources Centre

33 Robins Road
Tauranga
North Island
New Zealand

(075) 776085

Primary Personnel

Janice Priest, R.Kn., N.C., Dip herbology, H.Bt; also is editor of the national health magazine *Healthy Options* and is New Zealand's representative to the Bristol Cancer Help Centre, in England.

Directions

Two hours southeast of Auckland City. Along the coast, the centre is in Tauranga City.

Background

Herbal Education Resources Centre caters health classes in hospitals, educational institutions, community centres, and its own herbal centre. It offers a natural health clinic for treating all health-related problems, an herbal dispensary, a shop, and herbal gardens.

Illness Addressed

Cancer, all stages.

Types of Program Offered

Cancer diet, acupuncture, color therapy, meditation, herbal treatment, hypnotherapy, stress release, reflexology, and astrology-guided health charts. Individuals choose their own therapies. The centre's holistic approach to cancer is aimed at providing a better quality of life and a possible cure. For cases in which the cancer has advanced beyond chances for a cure, the centre promises a longer life span.

Costs

First consultancy, $25. Each subsequent appointment, $20.

Hippocrates Health Centre of Australia

Elaine Avenue
Mudgeeraba 4213
Gold Coast
Queensland
Australia

(075) 302860

Primary Personnel

Ronald Bradley, B.A., M.A., founding director.

Directions

Fly to Coolangatta or bus to Burleigh Heads. The centre is a 15-minute taxi ride from either place or a one-hour drive south of Brisbane.

Background

Hippocrates, the founder of medicine, long ago demonstrated that wholesome natural foods can restore and maintain vibrant health. The body cleans and regenerates itself. If you have the proper nutrients, you can enjoy a life free from illness and pain. The Hippocrates self-help program focuses on nutritional, physical, mental, and emotional balance and harmony.

Hippocrates Health Centre offers a complete health education, featuring Dr. Ann Wigmore's wheatgrass and living foods program, which, since 1960, has helped hundreds of thousands of people see that ideal health is natural for all of us. The program fosters regeneration, revitalization, and rejuvenation, leading to health, vigor, longevity, and youthful slimness.

Illness Addressed

Most health problems, including cancer, smoking, too much weight, and too much stress. However, students with contagious diseases may not attend.

Type of Program Offered

Dr. Wigmore's program offers a diet of 100% raw foods: sprouts, greens, fruits, vegetables, nuts, seeds, wheatgrass, and juices. It excludes all bread, flesh, dairy products, processed foods, and cooked foods. The curriculum features classes in gentle stretching exercises, wheatgrass, natural beauty care, massage, meditation, self-improvement, positive thinking, breathing, food combining, menu planning, weight loss, sprouting, dehydrating foods, goals and affirmations, relaxation, stress reduction, visualization, kitchen equipment, and permaculture. The centre's recreational facilities include a heated pool and spa, a tennis court, a steam room, bushwalking, rebounding, pingpong, and trampolining.

Related Readings

The Hippocrates Diet and Health Program by Dr. Ann Wigmore.

The Health Revolution by Ross Horne.

Improving on Pritikin by Ross Horne.

How I Conquered Cancer Naturally by Eydie Mae Hunsberger.

Length of Program/Stay

Minimum attendance is one week. Attendance of at least three weeks is strongly recommended.

Costs

Tuition fees are given in Australian, not United States, dollars and include a room with a private bath, all meals, educational instruction, a massage, a copy of Dr. Ann Wigmore's *The Hippocrates Diet and Health Program*, use of all recreational facilities, and a diploma. One week: $895 for a room shared with one other person, $1,195 for a private room. Two weeks: $1,695 for a room shared with one other person, $2,295 for a private room. Three weeks: $2,495 for a room shared with one other person, $3,395 for a private room.

Method of Payment

A deposit of half the tuition must be made in advance; the balance is paid upon arrival. Three credit cards are accepted: Bankcard, MasterCard, and Visa.

Medical Research Inc.

Severne Centre
Severne Street
Springlands
Blenheim
South Island
New Zealand

(03) 578–7335

Contact Person

Joy Breayley, Julia Davidson, Dale Yeoman.

Primary Personnel

Joy Breayley, Julia Davidson, Dale Yeoman.

Directions

Off Middle Renwick Road (the main highway to Nelson), look on the right at the second street past Springlands supermarket. The clinic is clearly signposted at the gates.

Background

Joy Breayley teaches meditation; Julia Davidson is a medical herbalist and nutritional counselor; Dale Yeoman conducts massage, teaching, and counseling. Together, they provide a holistic cancer treatment in conjunction with the patient's doctors. Medical Research is not a residential facility, but there are private accommodations close by.

Illness Addressed

Cancer.

Type of Program Offered

Herbal medicine, diet, lifestyle changes, enzymes, meditation, family counseling, visualization, relaxation, gentle massage, art therapy classes, group sessions, and herb teas served in the garden.

Costs

Costs not submitted for publication.

Radiant Health Centre

Doctors Hill/Goomalling Road
Northam
West Australia 6401
Australia

(096) 22 3427

Primary Personnel

Dorothea Snook, N.D., proprietor; Dr. Anna Shirage; Robert Pharnowhawk.

Background

The centre is an institute of natural healing and a private hospital for alternative medicines. It is situated on 24 acres of prime land, five minutes from the center of Northam. Approximately 15 acres are left in their natural state, providing the opportunity for bush walks. All rooms are private, and each set of two shares a toilet and bath. All guest rooms open onto the private swimming pool and patio, where patients may relax and soak up the healing rays of the sun. Supervision is provided 24 hours a day. Meals are served in the privacy of each room. Patients feeling up to it are invited to dine in the dining area and to socialize with other guests.

Upon arrival, each patient is examined by a qualified medical doctor who remains on call for the length of the patient's stay. The patient is billed privately by the doctor.

Radiant Health Centre is a member of ANTAB, the Australian Natural Therapies Accreditation Board.

Illness Addressed

Cancer and other degenerative diseases such as leukemia, arthritis, and AIDS. Also, asthma.

Type of Program Offered

Diets are worked out according to the needs of each patient. Saliva and urine tests are taken regularly. Juice therapy, sunshine therapy, breathing exercises, cold water therapy, physiotherapy, and colonics are administered as required. Iris diagnosis (iridology) and full body massage are provided for an additional fee. The only possible side effect is headaches.

Related Readings

What Way to Go by Dorothea Snook.

Length of Program/Stay

The average patient will stay for two weeks. More or less time may be spent, according to the patient's requirements. Outpatient treatment is available as a follow-up for all patients needing further care or for anybody not requiring 24-hour supervision.

Costs

Full-time care is $500 a person per seven-day week or $100 per day. Outpatient clinic is $25 per consultation (minimum of half an hour). Iridology is an additional $50, and a full body massage is $25 per treatment.

Method of Payment

Cash and checks are accepted. A list of participating private health funds will be provided upon application.

St. Columba's House

Woking
Surrey
England
United Kingdom

Contact Person

Vernon Templemore. Write to him at 50 The Kingsway, Ewell, Surrey KT17 1NA, England, or telephone him at 081–393–8145.

Directions

Woking is some 25 miles southwest of London and is easily reached by road and rail.

Background

Vernon Templemore is the Surrey regional representative of the Bristol Cancer Help Centre. He has been interested in healing for more than 20 years. Since retiring from the business world in 1986, he has devoted much of his time to holistic healing. He works mainly with cancer patients, lectures and teaches on the holistic approach to illness, and runs the St. Columba's House courses.

Illness Addressed

Cancer.

Type of Program Offered

Residential holistic healing courses for cancer patients, who may be accompanied by a relative or friend.

Length of Program/Stay

Three days for each course.

Related Readings

Let's Get the Fear Out of Cancer by Vernon Templemore. Gateway Books.

Costs

Costs not submitted for publication.

Hotaka Yojoen Holistic Health Center

7258–20 Ariake Hotaka-Cho
Minamiazumi-Gun
Nagano Prefecture 399–83
Japan

Telephone and *Fax*: (0263) 83–5260

Primary Personnel

Shunsaku Fukuda, founder.

Directions

From Shinjuku station, take the Chuo line to Matsumoto. Transfer to the Oito line at Matsumoto, and get off at Hotaka or Ariake. There are also trains directly to Hotaka, such as the Azusa limited express on the Chuo line. The center is a ten-minute taxi ride from Ariake or Hotaka. It is a three-hour train ride from Tokyo.

Background

This holistic health center is nestled on the slopes of the Japan Alps. The town of Hotaka is a rustic setting of hot springs, farms, pine trees, and honeysuckle. The center is three years old and has 24 tatami and Western-style accommodations.

Illness Addressed

Chronic diseases, including cancer.

Type of Program Offered

Macrobiotic natural whole foods diet, Onsen therapies (hand and foot germanium baths), natural hot spring baths, sauna baths with ultrared ray heat, herbal treatments, acupuncture, moxibustion, and Shiatsu massage. On occasion, there are musical concerts, workshops, and classes in ceramics, painting, and drawing.

Length of Program/Stay

One-week stay (minimum) is recommended, but a weekend is adequate if one has no other option.

Costs

Depends on length of stay.
Up to seven nights: 7,500 yen per night (includes two meals and use of Onsen).
From eight to 20 nights: 7,000 yen per night.
Long-term stay (more than 20 nights): 6,500 yen per night during summer season (April 16–October 14), 7,300 yen per night during winter season (October 15–April 15).
Initial acupuncture treatment with Onsen: 3,700 yen.
Outpatient Onsen therapy: 1,700 yen.

Support Groups

North America (Canada, United States)

Seymour M. Brenner, M.D.

Community Radiology Associates P.C.
2270 Kimball Street
Brooklyn, New York 11234
United States

(718) 253–6616
Fax: (718) 253–9833

Background

Dr. Brenner has been a practicing radiation oncologist for approximately 40 years. Five years ago, frustrated by a lack of progress in standard therapy for people dying from cancer, he began to investigate alternative methods. Dr. Brenner, convinced that the lives of many cancer victims can be saved by alternative therapies, hopes to win federal approval to conduct a scientific investigation into the effectiveness of alternative methods.

Type of Service Provided

Dr. Brenner acts as a consultant to cancer patients seeking information on the advisability of alternative vs. traditional methods of treatment. He offers advice and guidance as to what approach should be taken. He is in his office Mondays and Thursdays.

Costs

No charge for consultations. His advice is free. But if any work is actually performed (such as the taking of X-rays), the patient will be charged for that expense.

William M. Buchholz, M.D.
Susan W. Buchholz, Ph.D.

851 Fremont Avenue
Los Altos, California 94022
United States

(415) 948–3613

Primary Personnel

William M. Buchholz, M.D.; Susan W. Buchholz, Ph.D.

Directions

Follow highway 280 and exit at Magdelena Avenue east. Cross Foothill Boulevard and take an immediate right on Fremont. Go one-half mile to reach the office. Los Altos is between San Jose and Palo Alto.

Background

Dr. William Buchholz is an oncologist who works with his wife, Susan W. Buchholz, a clinical psychologist. William Buchholz, in practice since 1978, serves as a medical consultant to Cancer Support and Education (in Menlo Park, California), as well as to Commonweal Cancer Help Program (in Bolinas, California).

Illness Addressed

Cancer and general medical problems.

Type of Service Provided

Conventional and complementary therapy with an emphasis on imagery, psychological support, and development of strategies for dealing with cancer.

Related Readings

The Owner's Manual, A Guide for Owners of Human Bodies by William M. Buchholz, M.D. 1987.

Costs

Medical consultation: $195.
Office visit: $54.

Method of Payment

Cash and personal checks are accepted. Fees are generally covered by insurance.

Cancer Counseling Center of Ohio

1515 Lake Martin Drive
Kent, Ohio 44240
United States

(216) 922–1855
(216) 626–3115

Contact Person

Receptionist.

Primary Personnel

David G. Zimpfer, Ed.D., LPCC, NCC.

Directions

Located in a residential area just off state route 43, about four miles north of Kent. Easy access from Cleveland and Akron airports and from Ohio Turnpike.

Background

Treatment includes methods of Dr. Carl Simonton, Dr. Bernie Siegel, and the Voluntary Controls Program at Menninger Clinic. It proceeds on the assumption that cancer can be overcome and that the person with cancer can exert some control over the healing process. Illness may come to be seen as an opportunity for change or fulfillment. Quality of life is emphasized.

Bed and breakfast facilities on site are offered at nominal cost for persons who travel. Maps and lists of local motels and restaurants can be supplied.

Treatment is seen as complementary to any medical care being provided.

Illness Addressed

Cancer and other auto-immune diseases (e.g., rheumatoid arthritis, multiple sclerosis, lupus erythematosus, Sjogren's disease, Hashimoto's disease). Also other illnesses in which quality of life is affected or in which there is much anxiety.

Type of Service Provided

Biofeedback, guided imagery, psychosynthesis, meditation, relaxation and breathing, hypnosis, dreamwork, art therapy, and other methods are used as needed to promote optimal personal control and enhance immune functioning. Stress, pain, loneliness, helplessness, fatigue, and fatalism are dealt with. Counseling includes discussion of: the will to recover, death and dying, secondary gains of illness, stress factors, becoming an informed and assertive patient, taking responsibility for one's health, emotional issues that may aggravate the disease process, spirituality, resolution of interpersonal problems, love, and forgiveness. Exercise, nutrition, and continuation of personal productivity are emphasized, also.

Treatment is highly individualized and is conducted one-to-one. It is very helpful for a patient to have a partner, close friend, or loved one as a supporter. Such a person will be asked to attend at least some sessions.

Several times a year an intensive group therapy program is offered. Essentially the same treatment is provided as in individual work. The group program is especially useful for those who travel a long distance, for those who wish to reduce costs, and for those who desire the close interpersonal support that develops in a group. Support persons are encouraged to enroll and participate along with the client.

Related Readings

Cancer as a Turning Point by Lawrence LeShan. E.P. Dutton, 1989.

Getting Well Again by O. Carl Simonton, Stephanie Matthews-Simonton, and James Creighton. J.P. Tarcher, 1978.

Healing Yourself: A Step-by-Step Program for Better Health Through Imagery by Martin Rossman. Walker & Co., 1987.

Minding the Body, Mending the Mind by Joan Borysenko. Addison-Wesley, 1987.

Peace, Love, and Healing by Bernie Siegel. Harper & Row, 1989.

Books, audio tapes, and nutritional supplements are available through mail order. Catalog supplied upon request.

Length of Program/Stay

Clients who commute will generally have a two-hour session once or twice a week, depending on the level of anxiety and physical stamina. Treatment is arranged on a more frequent and intensive basis (several visits over two or three days or a full week) for those who come from a greater distance. Home visits can be arranged for people unable to travel.

Individual treatment most commonly extends for 25–30 hours. Upon evaluation, a decision is made whether to extend, to go on a reduced schedule of "booster" sessions, or to terminate.

Group therapy extends for a full-time week of five days.

Costs

$85 per hour of individual counseling. No additional fee for persons who accompany the client to individual counseling. Group therapy $995 per week. Reduced rate for support persons in group therapy.

Method of Payment

Cash, personal checks, and money orders are accepted. Most health insurance contracts cover at least some costs. Insurance claims can be filed on the client's behalf. In some cases, the insurance carrier can be billed directly for its contribution.

Payment for individual treatment is due upon completion of each session. Monthly billing is possible after financial responsibility has been established. Group therapy requires a $100 advance deposit to reserve a place; the balance is due at the start of the program.

Extended payment programs can sometimes be arranged.

Cancer Counselling Center

74 Sparkhall Avenue
Toronto, Ontario M4K 1G6
Canada

(416) 778–4567

Contact Person

Cole or Tucker.

Primary Personnel

M. Cole Cohen, Ph.D.; Tucker Feller, M.A.

Directions

Downtown Toronto.

Background

Based on the approach of Dr. O. Carl Simonton and other pioneers in psycho-social oncology, the program has evolved from the now generally accepted premise that beliefs, feelings, and lifestyle critically affect our health.

Illness Addressed

Cancer.

Type of Service Provided

Education and counseling for cancer fighters and their spouses or other support persons. Lifestyle analysis, individual counseling, and visualization coaching help participants learn to promote their own health. Emphasis is on emotional awareness, self-acceptance, and the role of social support. Each participant's response to the illness is explored in a safe, supportive atmosphere. Gentleness is of special importance.

Related Readings

Getting Well Again by Dr. O. Carl Simonton, Stephanie Matthews-Simonton, and James Creighton. J.P. Tarcher, 1978.

Love, Medicine, and Miracles by Dr. Bernie S. Siegel. Harper & Row, 1986.

Cancer as a Turning Point by Lawrence LeShan.

Length of Program/Stay

One week. Also, individual sessions as needed.

Costs

Costs, though not submitted for publication, are linked to the patient's income.

Method of Payment

Checks and cash are accepted. Some insurance companies will reimburse the patient.

Cancer Counselling Centre— Hope Program

2574 West Broadway
Vancouver, British Columbia V6K 2G1
Canada

(604) 732–3412

Contact Person

Moyra White, coordinator; Barbara Dams.

Directions

Located in the Kitsilano area of Vancouver. Closest major intersection is MacDonald Street and West Broadway.

Background

The Hope cancer program was founded in 1980 by Claude Dosdall and Moyra White. Both are cancer survivors. Since 1980, Hope has helped thousands of cancer patients and their families deal with the crisis of cancer away from the hospital environment. It is an intensive, structured, self-help cancer recovery program. Through Hope, cancer patients learn to take an active part in their fight for recovery. Hope believes a partnership between the cancer patient and the health professional is the only effective way to defeat cancer.

Illness Addressed

Cancer.

Type of Service Provided

It teaches techniques for stress reduction, relaxation, exercise, nutrition, visualization, and communication. Ongoing individual and group support assist the cancer patient and the family to deal effectively with the devastating physical and emotional effects of cancer and its treatments.

Related Readings

My God, I Thought You'd Died by Claude Dosdall and Joanne Broatch. Bantam-Seal Books, 1986.

Getting Well Again by O. Carl Simonton, M.D., Stephanie Matthews-Simonton, and James Creighton. J.P. Tarcher, 1978.

Length of Program/Stay

Workshops can run for one day, one evening, or a full weekend. Individual and family counseling can be ongoing.

Costs

Weekend seminar program costs $385 (Canadian) for two people—the cancer patient and a friend or relative.

Method of Payment

Cash and checks are accepted.

Cancer Support Community

401 Laurel Street
San Francisco, California 94118
United States

(415) 929–7400

Contact Persons/Primary Personnel

Victoria Wells, executive director; Ange Stephens, M.A., M.F.C.C.; Ricki Dienst, Ph.D.; Richard Cohen, M.D.; Ken Wilber; Allan Cohen, Ph.D.

Directions

This center is in the Laurel Heights area of San Francisco.

Background

This is a non-profit organization founded in 1986 by two women with cancer who, out of their own experience, created a community to meet the needs of people with cancer and the needs of families and friends. The entire staff has had cancer.

Illness Addressed

Cancer.

Type of Service Provided

Cancer Support Community offers understanding, support, and guidance to people with cancer and those who care about them. Its programs address the physical, mental, emotional, and spiritual needs of participants. Services include a variety of support groups for people with cancer, their families, and their friends; education programs (such as training and imagery, stress reduction, nutrition, and pain management); individual, couple, and family counseling; grief support; as well as library and referral services. Social activities (such as community parties and picnics) and volunteer opportunities occur regularly.

Costs

All programs are free. Donations are accepted.

Cancer Support and Education

(Creighton Health Institute)
1035 Pine Street
Menlo Park, California 94025
United States

(415) 327–6166 (call collect if necessary)

Primary Personnel

Karen Haas, M.A., director and former cancer patient; Carol Boeck, associate director and former cancer patient; Peggy Rogers, senior facilitator and former cancer patient.

Directions

Take highway 101. If coming from the north: exit at Marsh Road/Atherton. Turn left on Middlefield, right on Ravenswood, right on Pine. If coming from the south: exit at Willow Road/Menlo Park. Turn right on Middlefield, left on Ravenswood, right on Pine.

Background

Non-profit, tax-exempt organization provides in-depth support and psycho-social interventions. No medical treatment is provided at the center itself. Patients are strongly urged to bring a spouse, loved one, or other support person for no additional fee. The program is for children as well as adults.

Illness Addressed

Cancer, AIDS, chronic fatigue, and any other chronic or life-threatening illness.

Type of Service Provided

Step-by-step skills program teaches participants to take charge, handle stress, improve the quality of their lives, and maximize the effectiveness of chosen treatments, alternative or medical. Participants learn to live with commitment, become more effective fighters, and improve their psychological adjustment, regardless of the stage of illness.

The program is taught during 60 hours of group work and training, with each session lasting six hours. Participants may complete the program in two weeks or spread it out over ten. The program also includes options for individual sessions in massage; nutritional consultations; individual, couple, or family counseling; and a consultation with an internist/oncologist who believes people have a lot to do with their own recoveries. The group sessions are available weekdays from 9:30 a.m. to 4:30 p.m. Call the institute to learn the exact days involved.

Related Readings

Getting Well Again by O. Carl Simonton, M.D., Stephanie Matthews-Simonton, and James Creighton. J.P. Tarcher, 1978.

Love, Medicine, and Miracles by Bernie S. Siegel, M.D. Harper & Row, 1986.

Will to Live by Arnold Hutschnecker, M.D.

Costs

$2,400 for the full-service program (60 hours of group sessions, a consultation with an internist/oncologist, four counseling sessions, nine massages, and a nutritional consultation). Fee includes a spouse or other support person, who is not entitled to receive the massages.

$1,495 for the basic course (60 hours of group sessions, including a group nutritional presentation). Fee includes a spouse or other support person. Each service available in the full-service program may be purchased by basic course participants, on an à la carte basis, for a fee.

Center for Attitudinal Healing

19 Main Street
Tiberon, California 94920
United States

(415) 435–5022

Contact Person

Lynette Brohm, executive director.

Directions

North of San Francisco, take highway 101 north to the Tiberon Boulevard exit. Follow Tiberon Boulevard to the waterfront, turn right onto Main Street. The center is located on the bay side of the street near the Angel Island Ferry entrance.

Background

This center, founded in 1975 by Gerald Jampolsky, M.D., offers programs for children and adults with life-threatening or catastrophic illnesses. "For a child or an adult experiencing a catastrophic illness, there is a temptation to feel anger toward the world; alone, different, and isolated; that the universe is unloving and attacking. Healing begins when there is a shift in perception about an illness and its related problems. This shift in perception can occur as a child or an adult learns how to focus on helping others by extending only love, learns that each instant is the only time there is, and discovers that within that instant they do not perceive themselves as ill or in pain."

Illness Addressed

Cancer, AIDS, and any life-threatening illness.

Type of Service Provided

Attitudinal healing, acceptance, love, and support.

Living with Illness Group. For children ages 6–16 with life-threatening illnesses, their siblings, and those who have an ill parent. They learn they are not alone and are able to join others who truly understand.

Bereaved Children's Group. Children 6–16 meet to give and receive support as they share feelings about having lost a family member.

Young Adult's Group. Ages 16–26.

Adult Groups. Four groups for adults with serious illnesses and one for spouses and significant others.

The center has several groups for adults with life-threatening illnesses, including AIDS, breast cancer, etc. Other programs offered involve phone, person-to-person, and pen-pal communications to address long-term illness, loss, and grieving.

Related Readings

Love Is Letting Go of Fear by Gerald G. Jampolsky, M.D. Celestial Arts, 1979.

Teach Only Love by Gerald G. Jampolsky, M.D.

Goodbye to Guilt by Gerald G. Jampolsky, M.D.

Out of Darkness Into the Light by Gerald G. Jampolsky, M.D.

Love Is the Answer by Gerald G. Jampolsky, M.D., and Diane Cirincione.

One Person Can Make a Difference by Gerald G. Jampolsky, M.D.

Books and tapes are available through mail order.

Costs

All services are offered free of charge. Donations are accepted and encouraged.

Center for Cancer Survival

104 West Anapamu Street, Suite B
Santa Barbara, California 93101–3126
United States

(805) 962–6221

Contact Person

Richard Sheldon, founder.

Primary Personnel

Betty D. Sheldon, R.N., M.Ed., president; Barbara Kaplan-Winkler, Ph.D., clinical psychologist.

Directions

Located in the center of Santa Barbara, at the northwest corner of Anapamu Street and Chapala Street. Abundant free parking, well lighted, with easy handicap access.

Background

This is an independent, non-profit, non-medical, non-religious outreach educational program. It teaches members specific mental, emotional, and spiritual skills for survival on their journey to wellness and recovery from cancer. The benefits are not realized in the destination but in the journey itself. The focus is on attitudinal change and behavior modification. Adjuvant treatment choices are offered, without endorsement, to augment traditional cancer protocols. The center seeks members who want to create their future, not those who sit around worrying about it.

Illness Addressed

The main emphasis is on cancer; however, members with other life-threatening diseases may also benefit from the process.

Type of Service Provided

Training occurs in a series of six weekly two-hour sessions following a free introductory meeting. There are also monthly support groups. Lectures, discussions, speakers, audio- and video-tapes, films, demonstrations, role-playing, and handouts explore positive psychoneuro-immunological strategies.

Although all sessions take place in an environment not unlike a living room, this is a serious educational program requiring completion of homework assignments and a personal commitment to success. The training uses three major approaches: to encourage action and perhaps change the course of the illness; to provide an understanding of the illness, and through humor make the unacceptable bearable; and to reinforce positive mental attitudes while eliminating any negative resignation to a disastrous outcome. The center has a resource library of books, research papers, tapes, and films. Through exposure to these and other alternative options, members will assume control of their own treatment programs.

Related Readings

The works of Norman Cousins, Carl Simonton, Bernie Siegel, and Lawrence LeShan.

Costs

Support group meetings for members, graduates, and their families are free, by donation only. Costs for the education program not submitted for publication, but a sliding fee scale is available.

Method of Payment

Checks and cash are accepted. Insurance is accepted, but check with your company first.

Challenging Cancer

Group Meetings:
2223 Main Street, Suite 42
Seacliff Village Shopping Center
Huntington Beach, California 92648
United States

(714) 848–3473 (for more information)

Individual Counseling:
18275 Gum Tree Lane
Huntington Beach, California 92646
United States

(714) 848–3473 (for appointment)

Primary Personnel

Judith Sills, LCSW.

Directions

Seacliff Village Shopping Center is located in Huntington Beach at the intersection of Main Street and Yorktown.

Background

Judith Sills is a California state-licensed clinical social worker who received her master's degree in social work from the University of Houston and her bachelor of arts degree from the University of California, Los Angeles. She is a psychotherapist in private practice in Huntington Beach. She founded Challenging Cancer in January 1979.

Challenging Cancer is a self-help educational and support group for those with cancer and their family members. Anyone who has, or has had, cancer may attend, and group members are encouraged to bring a family member whenever possible. The methods learned at Challenging Cancer are not substitutes for medical treatment, but the skills, techniques, and knowledge gained can become a foundation for continued health improvement.

The group, which meets Thursday evenings from 7 to 9 p.m., concentrates on: teaching members to focus all their energy on improving their health; providing information on how persons with cancer can help themselves; informing members of literature, tapes, workshops, and community resources that can support their needs; relieving the isolation of the person with cancer and of their family; and having fun together.

Illness Addressed

Cancer.

Type of Service Provided

Psychotherapy (individual and group), imagery, relaxation, and wellness techniques.

Related Readings

Anatomy of an Illness by Norman Cousins. W.W. Norton and Co., 1979.

Getting Well Again by O. Carl Simonton, M.D., Stephanie Matthews-Simonton, and James Creighton. J.P. Tarcher, 1978.

Healing From Within by Dennis Jaffee.

Love, Medicine, and Miracles by Bernie S. Siegel, M.D. Harper & Row, 1986.

Peace, Love and Healing by Bernie S. Siegel, M.D.

Quantum Healing by Deepak Chopra.

The group will also furnish upon request information regarding past patients.

Costs

Donations.

Collaborative Medicine Center

10 Willow
Suite 4
Mill Valley, California 94941
United States

(415) 383–3197

Primary Personnel

Martin L. Rossman, M.D.

Directions

Mill Valley is a suburb north of San Francisco.

Background

This is not specifically a cancer treatment center, but it works with cancer patients by using a variety of supportive modalities. Emphasis is on helping people learn to support and activate their own healing processes.

Illness Addressed

Cancer and other diseases.

Type of Service Provided

Acupuncture, imagery, psychotherapy, relaxation, hypnosis, biofeedback, nutrition, Eastern medicine, body work, counseling, and massage.

Related Readings

Healing Yourself: A Step-by-Step Program for Better Health Through Imagery by Martin L. Rossman, M.D. Walker & Co., 1987.

Costs

Services range from $75 to $150 an hour.
Initial 90-minute interview with Dr. Rossman: $175.
Treatment plans are individualized.

Method of Payment

Cash, checks, Visa, and MasterCard are accepted. Fees are payable at time of service. Insurance may reimburse for some services.

Colorado Outward Bound School

945 Pennsylvania Avenue
Denver, Colorado 80203
United States

(303) 837–0880
(800) 477–2627
(303) 831–6956

Contact Person

Meg Ryan.

Directions

Colorado Outward Bound School's Leadville Mountain Center is a 2.5-hour drive west of Denver and is situated just outside of Leadville County, near Turquoise Lake.

Background

Started in 1961, Colorado Outward Bound is the nation's oldest wilderness adventure school. It promotes education, service, and personal growth through wilderness experience. While not a "survival" school in the literal sense, Outward Bound provides participants with the tools needed for success in the outdoors. Since 1985, it has been offering a course on "Challenging the Course of Cancer."

Illness Addressed

Cancer. (Any cancer patient or supportive partner may apply for admission; a physician's approval is required for acceptance.)

Type of Service Provided

Adjunct wilderness therapy for the psycho-social needs of those diagnosed with cancer and members of their families. A supportive group environment addresses the emotional, intellectual, and spiritual body as directly as medicine addresses the physical body. Sharing in the adventure of the wilderness and standing beside a supportive group of fellow "survivors" rewards participants in their quest for wholeness. Outward Bound activities may include: rock climbing, a ropes course, group problem-solving initiatives, trust-building exercises, and time spent alone in reflection. Course objectives include enhancing the wellness process, improving self-esteem, empowerment, and examining and affirming choice.

Length of Program/Stay

Challenging the Course of Cancer is a three-day course held in Leadville, Colorado at the Leadville Mountain Center. The course was scheduled four times in 1991.

Costs

Course is $240 plus a $50 application fee. Cost includes all camping equipment and outdoor clothing, food, instruction, and secondary insurance. There is no room fee; everyone sleeps outdoors. Some financial assistance is available. (A financial aid form will be included in your enrollment packet.)

Method of Payment

Cash and personal checks are accepted. Reservations over the telephone may be made with Visa or MasterCard. Before sending money, call the school and ask for an application.

Commonweal Cancer Help Program

P.O. Box 316
Bolinas, California 94924
United States

(415) 868–0970

Contact Person

Asoka Thomas, program coordinator.

Primary Personnel

Michael Lerner, Ph.D., president; Rachel Naomi Remen, M.D., medical director; Virginia Veach, Ph.D., M.F.C.C.

Directions

Please call first. From the Golden Gate Bridge, go approximately two and a half miles to Stinson Beach/Highway 1 exit. Continue about ten miles to Stinson Beach. Go five miles past town of Stinson Beach, take the first road to the left, just past the end of the lagoon. Make a left again at the end of this short connecting road and go about one mile. Turn left at the stop sign. Go half a mile, turn right on Mesa Road. Go approximately two and a quarter miles, enter driveway on left.

Background

Weeklong workshops take place roughly bimonthly, at the 60-acre Commonweal site in the Point Reyes National Seashore north of San Francisco. For developing the Commonweal Cancer Help Program, Dr. Lerner and Dr. Remen were awarded the first annual Gertrude Enelow Foundation Award for excellence in humanistic medicine by the Association for Humanistic Psychology in August 1986. Dr. Lerner is a former MacArthur Prize Fellow and is associated with the University of California, San Francisco, School of Medicine as a member of the adjunct faculty in the division of family and community medicine and as a policy fellow of the Institute for Health Policy Studies.

Illness Addressed

Cancer.

Type of Service Provided

Commonweal Cancer Help Program is an educational program, not a cancer therapy. It is designed to help participants reduce the stress of cancer, explore better health habits, be with others facing the same difficulties, and consider information on both established and complementary therapeutic options. The daily program includes support groups led by a trained psychologist, yoga and meditation, deep relaxation and imagery, massage therapy, work with sand trays, and healthy vegetarian meals. Participants must be under the care of an oncologist or other allopathic physician.

Related Readings

Varieties of Integral Cancer Therapies by Michael Lerner, $23 for fourth-class mail, $24.50 for first-class mail, free to workshop participants. (California residents need to add $1.26 for sales tax.) Also available are videotapes on the Bristol Cancer Help Centre in England, the Lukas Klinik in Switzerland, Dr. Hans Nieper in Germany, and Commonweal Cancer Help Program. The tapes are $22 for fourth-class mail, $23.50 for first-class mail. (California residents need to add $1.20 for sales tax.)

Costs

$1,080. Same fee for family member or other support person. Some scholarship support is available.

Method of Payment

Checks, MasterCard, and Visa are accepted.

Consciousness Research and Training Project Inc.

315 East 68th Street, Box 9G
New York, New York 10021
United States

Primary Personnel

Joyce Goodrich, Ph.D.

Background

This is a non-profit training and research project based on Dr. Lawrence LeShan's research and practice in meditation and healing.

Illness Addressed

Cancer and others, although illnesses are not addressed per se. Rather, the project establishes an environment in which the process of self-healing can take place as an adjunct to medical treatment.

Type of Service Provided

Five-day retreats and seminars are held around the country to train people to use the method. Occasionally, the project sends out a newsletter to those who have been trained. Applications and schedules for the training are available upon request.

Costs

$250 tuition for the five days. Room and board costs about $200.

Method of Payment

Checks and cash are accepted.

Exceptional Cancer Patients (ECaP)

1302 Chapel Street
New Haven, Connecticut 06511
United States

(203) 865–8392

Primary Personnel

Lynn Parrott, executive director; Susan Sperry, clinical director.

Background

Exceptional Cancer Patients, or ECaP, is a non-profit organization founded by Bernie Siegel, M.D., to provide group support for cancer patients. It is used as an adjunctive therapy; patients are urged to participate in their healing process.

Illness Addressed

Cancer, AIDS, and other chronic or life-threatening illnesses.

Type of Service Provided

Support groups, individual counseling, and workshops.

Related Readings

Getting Well Again by O. Carl Simonton, M.D., Stephanie Matthews-Simonton, and James Creighton. J.P. Tarcher, 1978.

Love Is Letting Go of Fear by Gerald G. Jampolsky, M.D. Celestial Arts, 1979.

Love, Medicine, and Miracles by Bernie S. Siegel, M.D. Harper & Row, 1986.

Peace, Love, and Healing by Bernie S. Siegel, M.D. Harper & Row.

You Can Fight for Your Life by Lawrence LeShan. M. Evans and Co., 1977.

Costs

Costs not submitted for publication, but a sliding fee scale is available. Mail-order books audio tapes, and videotapes are available. Free catalog sent upon request.

Healing Light Center Church

204 East Wilson
Glendale, California 91206
United States

(818) 244–8607

Primary Personnel

Rosalyn Bruyere, founder/director; Susan Brown, director of administration.

Directions

Centrally located in downtown Glendale near major freeways.

Background

This non-profit educational and religious organization deals with alternative health therapies and consciousness elevation, with a focus on ceremonial aspects.

Illness Addressed

Cancer, AIDS, and all other illnesses.

Type of Service Provided

Laying on of hands, healing, consultation with spirit guidance, healing church services, and seminary training.

Costs

Suggested donations: $30 per half hour, $50 per hour.

Method of Payment

Checks and cash are accepted. No credit cards are accepted. Insurance sometimes covers costs if the patient is referred by a physician.

Lawrence LeShan, Ph.D.

263 West End Avenue
New York, New York 10023
United States

Primary Personnel

Lawrence LeShan, Ph.D.

Background

Lawrence LeShan, an experimental psychologist, has spent four decades in research and psychotherapeutic work with cancer patients. He is generally considered a pioneer in dealing with emotional factors in the treatment of cancer.

Illness Treated

Cancer.

Type of Service Provided

Dr. LeShan will see people for a single consultation to evaluate their total situation. If appropriate, he will refer them and/or their families to specialists in psychotherapy.

Related Readings

Cancer as a Turning Point by Lawrence LeShan. Dutton, 1989.

Costs

Costs not submitted for publication but are based on a sliding scale.

Method of Payment

Cash and checks are accepted.

Life-Affirming Support Group

85 Aspinwall Road
P.O. Box 950
Briarcliff Manor, New York 10510
United States

(914) 941–8926

Primary Personnel

Pearl Bennette-Atkin, R.N., M.A., C.S.; Adam Atkin, Ph.D.

Directions

Groups meet in midtown Manhattan and Westchester County. Call for instructions.

Background

This support group is offered as an adjunct to traditional or alternative medical therapies. Whatever medical treatment you have had or are now having, a support group can help you to participate more actively in your own healing process and enhance your life through sharing with others.

Illness Addressed

Cancer and all life-threatening and/or chronic debilitating illnesses.

Type of Service Provided

Two weekly support groups; one meets in New York City, one in nearby Westchester County. Private consultations include psychotherapy, holistic health counseling, and lifestyle recommendations. Also relaxation, visual imagery work, and Shiatsu massage.

Related Readings

Love, Medicine and Miracles by Bernie S. Siegel, M.D. Harper & Row, 1986.

Healing Into Life and Death by Stephen Levine. Anchor/Doubleday, 1987.

You Can Heal Your Life by Louise Hay. Hay House, 1984.

Costs

Weekly support groups: No charge.
Private consultations (including psychotherapy, relaxation, and body work): $50–$75 per hour.

Method of Payment

Checks and cash are accepted.

Los Angeles Healing Arts Center

2211 Corinth Avenue
Suite 204
Los Angeles, California 90064
United States

(213) 477–8151

Primary Personnel

David E. Bresler, Ph.D., L.Ac., director of program development.

Directions

In west Los Angeles at the corner of Olympic and Corinth.

Background

Los Angeles Healing Arts is not a cancer treatment center, but it works with cancer patients by using supportive modalities. The emphasis is on helping people learn to support and enhance their own healing abilities.

Illness Addressed

Cancer, pain, stress, and other problems.

Type of Service Provided

Acupuncture, guided imagery, psychotherapy, counseling, relaxation training, stress management, hypnosis, biofeedback, nutritional and metabolic therapy, Hellerwork, chiropractic care, massage, and medical supervision.

Related Readings

Free Yourself From Pain by David E. Bresler, Ph.D. Simon and Schuster, 1979.

Costs

Each service carries its own fee, but costs not submitted for publication.

Method of Payment

Cash, personal checks, traveler's checks, money orders, Visa, and MasterCard are accepted.

Sandra McLanahan, M.D.

Route 1, Box 1680
Buckingham, Virginia 23921
United States

(804) 969—4680

Contact Person

Sandra McLanahan, M.D.

Directions

The clinic is at Yogaville, in Buckingham County, about one hour south of Charlottesville.

Background

Dr. McLanahan is the founder and primary physician of Integral Health Services, which was founded in 1974 as a therapeutic center for exploring multidimensional approaches to illness. The services include a chiropractor, massage persons, yoga instructors, and nutritional counselors. Programs offered are based on a spiritual approach to health and on the teachings of Swami Satchidananda. Dr. McLanahan also sees patients in Charlottesville.

Illness Addressed

Cancer, heart disease, and other chronic diseases.

Type of Service Provided

Allopathic medicine, individual nutritional programs, yoga classes, stress management, massage, homeopathy, guided imagery, visualization, counseling, psychospiritual approach, and group sessions.

Related Readings

"The Clinic Where Love and Medicine Go Hand in Hand," *Prevention*, 1977.

Costs

Individual sessions start at $85. Sliding scale and scholarships are available.

Method of Payment

Cash, traveler's checks, cashier's checks, and personal checks are accepted. Insurance generally covers physician costs.

New Hope Institute

500 Main Street
El Segundo, California 90245
United States

(213) 640–6605
Fax: (213) 322–5546

Contact Person

Barbara O'Hara.

Primary Personnel

Merlin D. Leach, D.C.H., Ph.D.

Directions

From Los Angeles International Airport, take Century Boulevard exit to Sepulveda, turn south to Imperial Highway West, go west three lights to Main Street, and turn south to the institute. Total distance from airport is about two miles.

Background

Dr. Leach is a board-certified and registered clinical hypnotherapist and hypno-anesthesiologist. He specializes in psychobiology and psychoneuro-immunology. He uses visualization and hypnosis to enhance other therapies and to improve the psychological condition of the patient. Hypnosis can be a very successful modality for managing pain without resorting to drugs.

Illness Addressed

Cancer. Also chronic and degenerative diseases.

Type of Service Provided

Counseling, hypnotherapy, hypno-analysis, hypno-anesthesia, and "state-dependent memory learning and behavior." Group sessions and individual sessions are available.

Costs

Group therapy: $15 to $30 per hour. Private therapy: $90 to $120 per hour. (A sliding scale is available for the needy.)

Method of Payment

Most insurances are accepted. Medicare and MediCal are not accepted.

Private Cancer Clinic Tours

P.O. Box 8254
Chula Vista, California 91912
United States

(619) 585–3926

Contact Person

Frankie Oviatt.

Directions

Chula Vista is eight miles from the border with Mexico. Tourists can be met either in Chula Vista or at their hotel or at the airport.

Type of Service Provided

Tour by private automobile of alternative therapy cancer clinics in or near Tijuana. Clinics and therapies are discussed on the way down to the border. The standard tour visits eight clinics: American Biologics, Bio-Medico (Hoxsey), Manner Clinic, Gerson, Hospital Ernesto Contreras, Immune Therapy Clinic, Santa Monica Hospital, and American Metabolics.

The tours are informal and without specific schedules. Tourists who wish to spend more time at one clinic than another, eliminate the visitation of those clinics in which they are not interested, or substitute a visit to a clinic not on the standard list may do so at no extra charge. The number of clinics visited depends on how long the tourist wishes to linger at each. The tourist may spend the entire tour at one clinic if he or she desires. Should you wish to see a doctor regarding your case, one is usually (but not always) available at each of the clinics. You may visit with patients, pick up brochures, and spend the time as you see fit.

Length of Program/Stay

The tour lasts up to eight hours, leaving Chula Vista at 8–9 a.m. and returning at 4–5 p.m. (There is no rebate for completing the tour in fewer than eight hours.) Tours are set up at least two days ahead of time, so call first. Tours are held Monday–Friday and in special circumstances on Saturday.

Costs

$125 per day per carload of people, for up to eight hours. (The car can hold up to five people besides the driver, but four or fewer are preferred.) The cost is per tour, not per clinic.

Psychosomatics

1729 Collingwood Drive
San Diego, California 92109
United States

(619) 272–9869

Primary Personnel

Dr. Robert Price.

Directions

Central San Diego, near the airport.

Background

Dr. Price has been working professionally in the mind-body field, also known as psychoneuro-immunology, for more than 20 years. His major training has been by Dr. Carl Simonton, Dr. Ernest Rossi, and Dr. Lawrence LeShan. He was research and clinical psychologist at Hospital Del Mar for eight years. He has lectured extensively in the mind-body field, and his television programs are shown on KPBS.

Illness Addressed

Cancer, arthritis, asthma, and cardiovascular problems. All psychosomatic disorders (disorders caused or merely aggravated by psychic and emotional processes).

Type of Service Provided

Psychotherapy and clinical hypnosis are the principal tools used in the psychoneuro-immuno-logical approach. Suggestions under hypnosis potentiate the normal healing response. The program consists of three 90-minute sessions spaced a day apart. Ericksonian hypnosis (a naturalistic hypnosis procedure) is taught. The specific disease and the psychological profile of the patient will determine how the period under hypnosis is used. The last session consists of a summing-up of factors that are seen to have contributed to and maintained the disease, followed by recommendations for changes that the patient can make to restore health. Audio tapes of the sessions are presented to the patient.

Related Readings

The Psychobiology of Mind-Body Healing by Dr. Ernest Rossi.

Mind-Body Therapy by Dr. Ernest Rossi and Dr. David Cheek.

Cancer as a Turning Point by Dr. Lawrence LeShan.

Peace, Love, and Healing by Dr. Bernie Siegel.

Costs

$75 for each 90-minute session.

Method of Payment

Cash and checks are accepted. Some insurance companies cover services. Champus (a national military insurance) is accepted.

Simonton Cancer Center

15601 Sunset Boulevard
Pacific Palisades, California 90272
United States

(213) 459–4434

Mailing Address:
P.O. Box 890
Pacific Palisades, California 90272
United States

Tape and Literature Department:
P.O. Box 1198
Azle, Texas 76020
United States

(817) 444–4073
(800) 338–2360

Contact Person

Admissions coordinator.

Primary Personnel

O. Carl Simonton, M.D.

Directions

Go to the end of Santa Monica Freeway (interstate 10). You will be on Pacific Coast Highway since the freeway ends there. From the end of the tunnel that puts you onto Pacific Coast Highway, it is three miles to the third signal, which is Temescal Canyon Road. Turn right, and go up the hill to Sunset Boulevard. Do not turn onto Sunset; drive straight onto the cancer center's grounds and continue until you reach a building that says "Welcome Presbyterian Conference Grounds." This is the retreat site.

Background

The "new patient" sessions last six days and are held once a month in Pacific Palisades, California, on 144 acres in the Santa Monica Mountains, 30 minutes from downtown Los Angeles and three minutes from the Pacific Ocean. Married patients must be accompanied by a spouse; singles are encouraged to bring a significant other. Each pair gets their own cabin and bath with "sparse but comfortable" furnishings.

Retreats are held in a summer-camp-type setting at the Presbyterian Conference Grounds in Pacific Palisades over the course of several days. They take a maximum of 14 patients and their support people.

Transportation from Los Angeles International Airport to the retreat can be provided by "Super Shuttle" or by taxi.

Illness Addressed

Cancer, although this method is applicable to all diseases of the immune system.

Type of Service Provided

This is an intensive group and individual psychotherapy program. Visualization, relaxation and mental imagery, goal setting, diet, and exercise are discussed. Topics include: stress, reconciling the issues of recovery and death, and secondary gains of illness. The program is designed to facilitate and enhance the treatment that patients are already receiving.

This program is based on the treatment module developed by O. Carl Simonton and Stephanie Simonton-Atchley 20 years ago in Fort Worth, Texas, where Dr. Simonton, a licensed radiation oncologist, was then practicing.

The program is strictly psycho-social. The only possible side effect is that some issues may be brought up that will make the patient desire further psychological or marital counseling.

Related Readings

Getting Well Again by O. Carl Simonton, M.D., Stephanie Matthews-Simonton, and James Creighton. J.P. Tarcher, 1978.

Love, Medicine, and Miracles by Bernie S. Siegel, M.D. Harper & Row, 1986.

Books and cassette tapes are available through mail order. The center will also furnish upon request information regarding past patients.

Costs

Six days of therapy cost $2,750. Meals and lodging for two cost $500. (The total cost is $3,250.) A nonrefundable deposit of $600 is due no later than one week prior to the session. The balance is due on the first day of the session.

Method of Payment

Personal, cashier's, and traveler's checks are accepted. The center encourages patients to bring their insurance forms. The center will help the patients fill out the forms in the hope they will be reimbursed. Check with your insurance agent to determine if your policy covers such treatment. It usually would be considered "outpatient psychotherapy."

Tour of Cancer Clinics

P.O. Box 4651
Modesto, California 95352
United States

(209) 529–4697 (1 p.m.–9 p.m.)

Primary Personnel

Frank Cousineau.

Background

The Cancer Control Society and Life Support sponsors this tour about six times a year. The tour visits the following alternative therapy clinics: Gerson Institute, Bio-Medical Center, Manner Clinic, Hospital Ernesto Contreras, American Biologics, Immune Therapy Clinic, American Metabolic Institute, and Hospital Santa Monica. The tour will initially leave from the Midtown Hilton, 400 North Vermont Avenue, Los Angeles at 7 a.m. It will then make three other pickups, the first at the Grand Hotel, One Hotel Way, Anaheim at 7:30 a.m.; the second at the Mission Bay Visitors Information Center, 2688 East Mission Bay Drive, San Diego at 9:15 a.m.; and the third at the Tourist Information Center, just over the border in Tijuana, Mexico, at 9:45 a.m. The tour will return to the Midtown Hilton around midnight. Tours have been given since May 1984.

Illness Addressed

Cancer, arthritis, multiple sclerosis.

Type of Service Provided

Bus tour of cancer clinics in Mexico.

Costs

The cost of the tour is $75 (tax deductible) a person regardless of the pickup point. Lunch will be provided at the Manner Clinic, and snacks will be available at the other clinics en route. The tour is also approved for ten hours of CE credits for nurses, who would pay $100.

Method of Payment

Send check at least seven days in advance, or pay in cash upon boarding the bus.

Wainwright House
Cancer Support Programs

260 Stuyvesant Avenue
Rye, New York 10580
United States

(914) 967–6080

Contact Person

Richard Grossman, program director.

Primary Personnel

Julie Butler; Rachel Gluckstein, R.N.; Richard Grossman; Mary Zachary, M.D.

Directions

Rye is a regularly scheduled stop on Metro North Railroad. By car, take highway I-95 to exit 19 (Playland Parkway), make a right turn at the first light on Playland Parkway, onto Milton Road. At the second light (flashing yellow) turn left onto Stuyvesant Avenue. After half a mile, Wainwright House is on the right.

Background

Weeklong residential retreats are offered four or five times a year on the grounds of Wainwright House, a non-profit, nonsectarian educational conference center on the shore of Long Island Sound, overlooking Milton Harbor. Wainwright House Cancer Support Programs are based on the Commonweal Cancer Help Program.

Illness Addressed

Cancer.

Type of Service Provided

Wainwright House is not a cancer therapy. It is devoted to patient education, health promotion, and stress management. It is designed to help those with cancer achieve increased autonomy, manage pain, ameliorate anxiety and depression, engage in effective life planning, and make informed choices among conventional and complementary therapies. The program includes yoga and meditation, relaxation and mental imagery training, massage therapy, nutritional counseling, and personal expression through art, poetry, music, and movement. Nondairy vegetarian meals are served. Participants must be under the care of an oncologist or other physician.

Costs

$1,000. Scholarship funds are available for those in financial need.

Wellness Community

2190 Colorado Avenue
Santa Monica, California 90404–3506
United States

(213) 453–2300
Fax: (213) 315–9854

Primary Personnel

Harold H. Benjamin, Ph.D., founder and president.

Background

The primary purpose is to make it possible for people with cancer to learn that they can be active participants in the fight for recovery and are not relegated to being hopeless, helpless, passive victims of the illness. Wellness Community is in support of and in addition to traditional medical treatment.

Wellness Community is a non-profit organization.

Illness Addressed

Cancer.

Type of Service Provided

The organization offers lectures and presentations to cancer patients and their families; it teaches stress management, relaxation, pain control, nutrition, and biofeedback; and it provides ongoing weekly psychotherapeutic groups led by licensed facilitators. Groups at which people with cancer can learn about the services offered meet Tuesday evenings from 7 p.m. to 9 p.m. and Fridays from 11 a.m. to 1 p.m. Monthly calendars of gatherings and speakers are available.

Costs

There is no charge for services provided.

Its national headquarters is in Santa Monica, California, but the Wellness Community can also be contacted at its several other locations (all in the United States):

109 West Torrance Boulevard, #100
Redondo Beach, California 90277
(213) 376–3550

3760 Convoy Street, #320
San Diego, California 92111
(619) 467–1065

1844 Terrace Avenue
Knoxville, Tennessee 37916
(615) 546–4661

131 North County Line Road
Hinsdale, Illinois 60521
(708) 323–5150

1924 East Glenwood Place
Santa Ana, California 92705
(714) 258–1210

100 North Hill Avenue, #107
Pasadena, California 91106
(818) 796–1083

350 North Wiget Lane, #101
Walnut Creek, California 94598
(415) 933–0107

Towers of Kenwood
8044 Montgomery Road, #385
Cincinnati, Ohio 45236
(513) 791–4060

299 West Hillcrest Drive, #220C
Thousand Oaks, California 91360
(805) 494–6406

1146 Beacon Street
Brookline, Massachusetts 02146
(617) 232–2300

P.O. Box 232
Millersville, Maryland 21108
(301) 987–9299

Wellness Response Center

610 Anacapa Street
Santa Barbara, California 93101–1615
United States

(805) 963–1661

Primary Personnel

Charles J. Lynch, M.F.C.C.

Background

Wellness Response Center, sponsored by the Institute of Behavioral Medicine (a California non-profit corporation), offers informal drop-in groups for people who have or have had cancer and for their families and friends. The center was organized to provide people with new tools for confronting the crises associated with cancer. Its primary purpose is to teach people to mobilize their strengths and "will to live" in support of overall treatment. The Wellness Response Center program is in support of and in addition to regular medical treatment.

Illness Addressed

Cancer and other life-threatening diseases.

Type of Service Provided

The Sharing and Caring Group offers its members the chance to explore with others the methods they have used to enhance the quality of their lives, as well as providing an opportunity to form friendships and mutual support networks for learning to attain a high level of wellness and for living life to its fullest. The patients and/or their significant others may attend as often as they wish, without obligation of any kind. Other services offered are biofeedback, hypnosis, counseling (individual, couple, and family), and training in imagery and visualization.

Costs

Sharing and Caring Group is free. Other services entail a fee on a sliding scale.

Wellspring Center for Life Enhancement

3 Otis Street
Watertown, Massachusetts 02172
United States

(617) 924–8515

Primary Personnel

Joan Klagsbrun, Ph.D., and Connie Lorman, Ed.D., co-directors.

Directions

Watertown is a suburb of Boston.

Background

Wellspring Center for Life Enhancement offers psychological, social, and spiritual support to individuals and families with cancer and other life-threatening diseases. The programs are designed to complement, not replace, any ongoing medical treatment the patients are receiving. The techniques and practices are based on studies of how the mind affects the body.

Illness Addressed

Cancer and other life-threatening diseases.

Type of Service Provided

Small support groups (8–12 participants) are led by skilled facilitators. There are support groups for people with cancer and separate groups for family and friends. Intensive weekend workshops, consultations, referrals, training, and a resource library are also offered. The focus is on exploring feelings, giving and receiving support, and learning life-enhancing relaxation techniques such as stress reduction, meditation, and visualization. There is also a visitor's program in which trained volunteers visit people at home or in the hospital.

Costs

Fees are on a sliding scale and range up to $300 for a ten-session support group. No one is turned away for lack of funds. There is no charge for the visiting volunteers.

Method of Payment

Insurance companies generally reimburse participants for the cost.

Support Groups

Overseas (Australia, Japan, United Kingdom)

Cancer Support Association Inc.

80 Railway Street
Cottesloe (Perth)
Western Australia 6011
Australia

(09) 384 3674
(09) 384 4556

Contact Person

Leslie or Gary.

Primary Personnel

Cath Meaden, president; Ellen Levett, secretary; Kaye Murray, treasurer; Leslie Burke, office manager; Gary Elsberry, administration and public relations manager; Lisa Campbell, counselor.

Directions

The association is located in Cottesloe, a suburb of Perth, the capital city of the state of Western Australia.

Background

The Cancer Support Association was formed and incorporated in 1984. Its aims and objectives are to assist cancer patients and their families; to engage in public education programs for cancer patients and their families, colleagues, and friends to improve the quality and length of life for the cancer patient in a manner both complementary and supplementary to prescribed medical treatments; to provide active support for cancer patients and their families to help them recognize the importance of their personal contribution in fighting and overcoming cancer; and to encourage those with cancer to accept responsibility for the quality of their lives by paying particular attention to the holistic approach of self-care, which includes meditation, positive thinking, diet and nutrition, and related subjects.

Type of Service Provided

Emotional and psychological counseling, meditation, Tai Chi, massage, and access to a large resource library containing information on all types of cancer treatments.

Costs

The association is a non-profit organization. All income—derived from private voluntary donations, government grants, and bequests—is strictly applied toward fulfilling the association's aims and objectives.

Cheltenham Cancer Help Centre

14 Clarence Square
Cheltenham, Gloucestershire GL50.4JN
England
United Kingdom

(011) 44–242–525437

Primary Personnel

Richard Lamerton, M.D., Hospice of the Marches.

Directions

Take exit 10 or 11 from M5.

Background

Cheltenham Cancer Help Centre is under the auspices of the Hospice of the Marches. For terminally ill patients, there is no discontinuity of care. This is not an inpatient facility. The staff visits people's homes as often as necessary. The clinic is open every other Saturday.

Illness Addressed

Cancer, AIDS, leukemia, and amyotrophic lateral sclerosis.

Type of Service Provided

They give advice on diet and nutrition; provide a personal interview with a counselor; and use healing and relaxation techniques such as acupuncture, massage, osteopathy, yoga, counseling, hypnotherapy, art therapy, and conventional therapy.

Related Readings

The clinic will provide upon request information regarding past patients.

Costs

A day's care in one of the clinics costs about 50 pounds per patient. This includes therapist's fees, the Bristol Diet lunch, and rent of the building. However, no payment is required. Funds are raised by appeals, street collections, garage sales, etc. Patients may make a voluntary donation.

Chiltern Cancer Counselling

193 Tring Road
Aylesbury
Buckinghamshire HP20 1JH
England
United Kingdom

(0296) 24854

Contact Person

Joyce Parsons.

Primary Personnel

Joyce Parsons, RGN, SCM, DHP, MNAHP.

Directions

About one mile from Aylesbury town center on the A41 Aylesbury–Watford–London road.

Background

Chiltern Cancer Counselling was founded in 1984 to meet the needs of cancer patients and their families by offering a holistic program for use alongside orthodox medical treatment.

Illness Addressed

Cancer.

Type of Service Provided

Chiltern Cancer Counselling offers a holistic healing program; helps dispel the fear associated with the disease and the word "cancer"; directs effort toward the cause of the disease; encourages a new, positive approach using group therapy; and provides a supportive link for cancer patients and their families.

Group therapy sessions include work with psychotherapy, biofeedback, meditation, relaxation, visual imagery, and healing.

Costs

30 pounds per consultation.

Method of Payment

Personal checks and cash are accepted.

Hereford Cancer Help Clinic

Brookfield
Tarrington
Herefordshire HR1.4HZ
England
United Kingdom

(011) 44–432–890341

Primary Personnel

Richard Lamerton, M.D., Hospice of the Marches.

Directions

Exit 2 from M50. A417 to Ledbury. A438 (Hereford Road) to Tarrington.

Background

Hereford Cancer Help Clinic is under the auspices of the Hospice of the Marches. For terminally ill patients, there is no discontinuity of care. This is not an inpatient facility. The staff visits people's homes as often as necessary. The clinic is open every Friday.

Illness Addressed

Cancer, AIDS, leukemia, amyotrophic lateral sclerosis, Parkinson's disease, etc.

Type of Service Provided

They give advice on diet and nutrition; provide a personal interview with a counselor; and use healing and relaxation techniques such as acupuncture, massage, osteopathy, yoga, art therapy, counseling, hypnotherapy, and conventional therapy.

Related Readings

The clinic will provide upon request information regarding past patients.

Costs

A day's care in one of the clinics costs about 50 pounds per patient. This includes therapist's fees, the Bristol Diet lunch, and rent of the building. However, no payment is required. Funds are raised by appeals, street collections, garage sales, etc. Patients may make a voluntary donation.

Institute for Religious Psychology

4–11–7 Inokashira
Mitaka-shi
Tokyo 181
Japan
0422–48–3535

Contact Person

Yujiro Shimogori, coordinator and chief of administration.

Primary Personnel

Dr. Hiroshi Motoyama, Shinto priest, as well as founder and head priest of the Tamamitsu Shrine.

Background

Dr. Motoyama is a worldwide lecturer with interests in religion, parapsychology, science, and holistic health. His inventions include: a machine that measures the functional conditions of meridians and their corresponding internal organs; and a machine that measures changes in the electromagnetic field surrounding the body.

The institute seeks to stimulate, strengthen, and support physical, mental, and spiritual health and to promote synchronicity between body, mind, and spirit.

Type of Service Provided

Acupuncture, to restore a balanced flow of energy in the body; Kundalini yoga, to progress to a higher state of consciousness; exercises that regulate the balanced flow of energy in the body; meditation, to reduce stress; karma and reincarnation studies, to examine related factors and chronic and degenerative diseases that may have manifested themselves in the patient's previous lifetimes (and thus possibly affect the patient's psychological profile); and spiritual consultations, but only when a crisis condition warrants such intervention.

Costs

Costs not submitted for publication.

LIFE Cancer Centre

Maristowe House
Dover Street
Bilston, West Midlands
WV14.6AL
England
United Kingdom

0902–409164

15 Holyhead Road
Upper Bangor
North Wales
United Kingdom

0248–370076

Primary Personnel

Dr. M.C. Patel, founder; Chris Barrington, Sian Edwards, and Rita Goswami, directors.

Background

There is increasing evidence that cancer is related to the way that people live their lives. Independent research has shown that cancer can be prevented by the right mental approach to life and in a large number of cases can be cured by a change in lifestyle. In all cases, quality of life can be improved. Cancer is related to the stress of living in the "rat race," the conditions of the environment people live in, the foods they choose to eat, and the air they breathe. Many members of the medical profession believe preventive measures are the only way of solving the world's cancer problem.

LIFE is a group of people dedicated to helping the sufferers of cancer. The staff has long-standing experience in the teaching of techniques of relaxation and self-awareness and in the application of complementary techniques for the well-being of body, mind, and spirit.

Illness Addressed

Cancer.

Type of Service Provided

Advice and support for all cancer sufferers, including children, and therapy complementing orthodox allopathic treatment to help the cancer patient fight for recovery. Therapies include yoga, meditation, visualization, psychotherapy, biofeedback, affirmation, Shiatsu massage, reflexology, Bach flower remedies, holistic diet, etc. The centre also provides a counseling service to help families come to terms with cancer.

Costs

Costs not submitted for publication.

Meditation for Cancer Patients

50 Garnet Street
Dulwich Hill
New South Wales 2203
Australia

(02) 559 5666

Primary Personnel

Chris Magarey, M.D., assistant professor.

Directions

By Car: New Canterbury Road from Sydney—about 20 minutes. Turn left at Garnet Street at Hurlstone Park.
By Train: Bankstown line from Sydney—about 20 minutes. Exit at Hurlstone Park. It's then a five-minute walk.

Background

Dr. Magarey is a cancer surgeon and research worker. He studies psychological factors in the resistance of patients to their own cancer. There is a focus on the value of meditation for cancer patients and for their relatives and friends.

Illness Addressed

Cancer, AIDS, and any health or stress problem.

Type of Service Provided

Siddha meditation practice and philosophy is taught in a small-group course that includes clinical opinion regarding cancer management and meditation. Free introductory lecture and instruction is available. Additionally, it offers education to health workers in the healing process. Evening programs and courses are available.

Related Readings

A large selection of titles about Siddha meditation is available. Relaxation, meditation, and chanting tapes are also available.

Length of Program/Stay

Six weeks, two hours a week. Follow-up activities are available.

Costs

Six-week course in meditation: $90 (Australian).
Other evening programs are free.

Method of Payment

Cash, checks, and money orders are accepted.

Newark Cancer Help Group

Woods Court
Newark
Nottinghamshire
London
England
United Kingdom

703–274
525–655

Contact Person

Mr. Gerry Martin, chairman.

Background

This is a caring group offering therapies that treat the whole person and that are complementary to orthodox medical treatments.

Illness Addressed

Cancer.

Type of Service Provided

The group meets at 7:30 p.m. on the second and fourth Monday every month. In attendance are nurses, nursing sisters, dietitians, and a reflexologist. The services of a hypnotherapist are also available. There is group and individual counseling for patients and for those who care for them. The group will make hospital visits, if required, and will help where needed, such as with medications and vitamins.

Costs

All services are free.

Plymouth Natural Health and Healing Centre

100 Lipson Road
Lipson
Plymouth
Devon PL4 8RJ
England
United Kingdom

Plymouth 228785
Plymouth 660712
Cornwood 383

Primary Personnel

Dr. Alec Forbes, president; Dr. Adrian White, vice president; Frank Smale, vice president.

Background

Founded in 1977, the centre is a registered charity affiliated with Bristol Cancer Help Centre, National Federation of Spiritual Healers, LIFE Cancer Centre, and LIFE Foundation. Its aim is to help people help themselves. It is staffed entirely by volunteers. The centre is open Monday–Friday from 11 a.m. to 4 p.m.

Illness Addressed

Cancer and any other form of ill health.

Type of Service Provided

Counseling, healing, relaxation, visualization, meditation, reflexology, yoga, osteopathy, homeopathy, Shiatsu massage, and nutritional advice. Patients learn how to release and mobilize inner resources of self-healing.

Costs

Donation.

"Ray of Light" Spiritual Healing Centre

25 Hough Green
Ashley, Altrincham
Cheshire WA15 0QS
England
United Kingdom

061–928–4566

Contact Person

Raymond C. Gardner, administrator.

Primary Personnel

Ramond C. Gardner, DSNU; Mrs. J. Gardner, DSNU; Mrs. M. Stoba; Mr. A. Froude; Mrs. J. Castelli.

Directions

Altrincham Cheshire Library, opposite the Altrincham bus station and railway station.

Background

Ray of Light was founded in 1975. Healing sessions are held every Wednesday morning from 9:45 a.m. to 12:15 p.m. Patients can come in any time between those hours. Appointments are not necessary, because the waiting time is not long (at most 30 minutes and usually no more than 10).

Illness Addressed

The centre believes that every disease or injury responds to spiritual healing, either by more refreshing sleep, an easement of pain, or a general uplifted feeling of well-being. Although instantaneous cures have occurred, they are not the general rule. Healing builds up week by week.

Type of Service Provided

After the patient has explained the problem, healing commences with the laying on of hands and quiet prayer. Treatment after the first session takes about 10 minutes.

Costs

No fees. No charge for treatment. But there is a free-will donation box for people who wish to help cover the cost of running the centre and renting the room.

Relaxation Centre of Queensland

Corner of Brookes and Wickham Streets
Fortitude Valley
Brisbane 4006
Queensland
Australia

07 854–1986
Fax: 7–2524157

Contact Person

Marge Garrett or Lionel Fifield.

Primary Personnel

Lionel Fifield.

Directions

One mile from the center of Brisbane.

Background

Many doctors, psychiatrists, naturopaths, and other therapists recommend the Relaxation Centre as part of a program toward regaining health or coping with an ongoing illness.

Type of Service Provided

A program of more than 50 ways to help people relax, find a deeper personal peace, build a lifestyle, and enhance their self-esteem.

Related Readings

The centre publishes a newsletter every two months.

Costs

Newsletter is free. Other costs not submitted for publication.

Thorpe Bay Self-Help Cancer Group

22 St. James Avenue
Thorpe Bay
Southend-on-Sea
Essex SS1 3LH
England
United Kingdom

(0702) 584111
(0702) 587640

Contact Person

Angela Ekers or Maureen Holmes.

Primary Personnel

Angela Ekers.

Background

The group's aim is to give support to people who have cancer and to their families. Angela Ekers is a member of the National Federation of Spiritual Healers Association. The group is registered with Bacup and CancerLink.

Illness Addressed

Cancer.

Type of Service Provided

The group meets in an informal atmosphere every Friday at 7 p.m. The group provides: a way for sharing problems and information; the teaching of relaxation, meditation, and positive thinking; the use of a library with books and tapes; art therapy; dietary help; refreshments; a way to make new friends; and, if desired, spiritual healing.

Costs

Costs not submitted for publication.

Information Services

North America (Canada, United States)

Arlin J. Brown Information Center Inc.

P.O. Box 251
Fort Belvoir, Virginia 22060
United States

(703) 752–9511

Directions

Mail and phone only.

Background

Founded in February 1963 as an information organization, the Arlin Brown Center investigates nontoxic cancer therapies. It publishes a newsletter that includes questions and answers with leading specialists. This group also has proposed a national health freedom bill to allow Americans to use any type of remedy they choose. The center was the first cancer organization in the United States devoted to nontoxic treatments. This is an information center only.

Type of Information Offered

Information on different types of cancer, health methods, degenerative diseases, and nontoxic cancer therapies.

Related Readings

March of Truth on Cancer.

Health Victory Bulletin. Monthly newsletter.

The center also offers a mail-order book list upon request.

Costs

Member for one year: $25.
Contributing member for one year: $35.
Supporting member for two years: $80.
Supporting member for five years: $200.
Life member: $500.
Perpetual member: $1,000.

Method of Payment

Cash and checks are accepted.

Cancer Control Society and Cancer Book House

2043 North Berendo Street
Los Angeles, California 90027
United States

(213) 663–7801

Contact Person

Lorraine Rosenthal.

Directions

Interstate 5 to Los Feliz off ramp. Go west for about one mile to North Berendo, turn left, and go one and a half blocks. Or else take Hollywood Freeway (101) to Vermont off ramp, go north about one and a half miles to Franklin, turn left, then go two blocks to North Berendo and turn right.

Background

This is an informational and educational non-profit organization. The Cancer Control Society Convention, held in Los Angeles during the Labor Day weekend, has been the largest gathering of its kind for almost 20 years.

Illness Addressed

Cancer. It will also direct patients to clinics that offer treatment for arthritis, heart problems, and multiple sclerosis.

Type of Information Offered

An information set, films, books, videos, a clinic directory, a list of clinic tours, and lists of patients. It also offers a bookstore that has a comprehensive mail-order list; conventions; and the *Cancer Control Journal*, which it publishes.

Related Readings

An extensive list is available of books and reprints on cancer and other nutrition-related diseases. Films and videos are also available.

Costs

Yearly membership: $25.
Information set (doctor and clinic lists, patient lists, book house list, clinic flyers, membership application, other): $5.
Information set plus a sample issue of *Cancer Control Journal*: $10.

Method of Payment

Money orders and checks are accepted.

Cancer Federation

P.O. Box 52109
Riverside, California 92517–3109
United States

(714) 682–7989

Primary Personnel

John Steinbacher, executive director.

Background

Cancer Federation is a non-profit organization that funds cancer immunology research and scholarships for such schools as San Jose State, Chico State, the University of California at Santa Barbara, and the University of Oregon. It receives 95% of its income from the collection and resale of discards. Some of its income comes from membership dues.

Illness Addressed

Cancer.

Type of Information Offered

The federation publishes a quarterly magazine, holds free meetings, counsels cancer patients and their families, and maintains a lending library of materials on the latest immunological therapies. Patients are referred to medical centers and/or physicians in the United States who employ immunology as a primary therapy. Cancer Federation members receive a subscription to the group's magazine, as well as free books, tapes, monographs, and other material.

Costs

Membership is $20 a year. All donations are tax deductible.

Method of Payment

Checks and money orders are accepted.

CanHelp

3111 Paradise Bay Road
Port Ludlow, Washington 98365–9771
United States

(206) 437–2291

Primary Personnel

Patrick M. McGrady Jr., founder and director; Dorris Stellner, assistant director.

Background

Mr. McGrady is a medical writer with a talent for translating medical jargon into plain English. A former *Newsweek* Moscow bureau chief, he wrote *The Youth Doctors* and *The Love Doctors* and co-authored *The Pritikin Program for Diet & Exercise* and *Life Zones*. He founded CanHelp to provide clients with up-to-date information on both conventional and alternative therapies. He is not a doctor and does not prescribe therapies. Call first, or send a stamped, self-addressed envelope for free literature.

Illness Addressed

Cancer.

Type of Information Offered

After analyzing the patient's medical records and questions and consulting with its own specialists, CanHelp writes an evaluative and detailed report on those alternative, orthodox, and experimental therapies that would appear to offer its client the most promise. The report (5–15 pages) covers such matters as content of treatment, length of stay, location, quality of care, costs, phone numbers, personality of physician, and caveats, if any. Accompanying the report are background articles about recommended physicians and treatments and up-to-date computer printouts of relevant studies from CancerLit and other computer medical databases. CanHelp also answers brief follow-up questions and assists in solving logistical problems. The service is available seven days a week, 24 hours a day. Reports are sent by express mail, usually within seven working days of receipt of medical records. In emergencies, reports can be completed in as few as two days and sent to the client via fax or modem.

Costs

$400 for seven-day personal report.
$500 for foreign-based client's personal report.
$150 extra for emergency two-day personal report.

Method of Payment

A check made to "CanHelp" should be sent with the medical records.

Center for Science in the Public Interest

1875 Connecticut Avenue N.W.
Suite 300
Washington, D.C. 20009–5728
United States

(202) 332–9110
Fax: (202) 265–4954

Contact Person

Publications department or nutrition department.

Directions

Take the Washington Metro subway's Red line to the Dupont Circle stop, use the Q Street exit, go three blocks up Connecticut Avenue to the intersection of Connecticut Avenue and T Street, just before the Washington Hilton hotel. The center is in the Universal North building.

Background

Center for Science in the Public Interest (CSPI) is the nation's leading consumer group concerned with food and nutrition issues. CSPI focuses on diseases that result from consuming too many calories; too much fat, sodium, and sugar; and not enough fiber. CSPI has 250,000 members.

Illness Addressed

Cancer and heart disease.

Type of Information Offered

All CSPI members receive the *Nutrition Action Healthletter*, which takes a self-help and consumer advocacy perspective to address the prevention of cancer and heart disease. Other publications include the Anti-Cancer Eating Guide poster and the Chemical Cuisine poster on food additives. A publication list will be sent on request.

Costs

Membership for one year is $19.95 for United States residents and $27.95 for everyone else. Membership includes a subscription to *Nutrition Action Healthletter* (published 10 times a year), a membership package including posters, and a 10% discount on the purchase of various publications.

Method of Payment

Personal checks, money orders, Visa, and MasterCard are accepted on United States orders. Visa, MasterCard, and postal orders (in United States funds) are the only methods accepted on foreign orders.

Committee for Freedom of Choice in Medicine Inc.

1180 Walnut Avenue
Chula Vista, California 91911
United States

(619) 429–8200

Primary Personnel

Robert Bradford; Michael Culbert.

Background

This is a lobbying group that publishes a quarterly newsmagazine called *The Choice*, as well as special reports. This group is headed by people in charge of American Biologics Hospital, in Tijuana, Mexico. It is the successor to the Committee for Freedom of Choice in Cancer Therapy Inc., which was formed in 1974.

Illness Addressed

Chronic systemic metabolic dysfunctions.

Type of Information Offered

The Choice, a quarterly newsmagazine; mail-order supplements; and special reports.

Costs

$16 for a one-year subscription.

Method of Payment

Cash, checks, American Express, Discover, MasterCard, Visa, and money orders are accepted.

Foundation for Advancement in Cancer Therapy (FACT)

P.O. Box 1242
Old Chelsea Station
New York, New York 10113
United States

(212) 741–2790

P.O. Box 215
200 East Lancaster Avenue
Wynnwood, Pennsylvania 19096
United States

(215) 642–4810

Contact Person

Ruth Sackman.

Background

This non-profit educational organization distributes information on cancer prevention and nontoxic therapies for cancer. Its headquarters is in New York, with another chapter near Philadelphia.

Illness Addressed

Cancer.

Type of Information Offered

FACT believes in the "total person approach," which involves early noninvasive diagnosis, nutrition, detoxification, structural balance, and therapies involving the mind-body connection. Some types of therapy are fever, immuno, cellular, and botanical.

Related Readings

Mail-order books, articles, and cassette tapes are available.

Costs

Any contribution is accepted. For $10 a year, you will receive a subscription to *Cancer Forum*, a FACT publication.

Method of Payment

Cash, checks, and money orders are accepted.

Health Resource

209 Katherine Drive
Conway, Arkansas 72032
United States

(501) 329–5272
Fax: (501) 329–8700

Primary Personnel

Janice Guthrie.

Background

Janice Guthrie is a cancer patient who researched her rare type of cancer in medical center, public, and university libraries. With the information she gathered, she was able to find a specialist who had done research on her particular tumor, and thus she was able to be an active participant in the decisions regarding her own treatment. Her research helped her gain control over her personal health, and she decided to perform the same research as a service for other people with medical problems.

Illness Addressed

Cancer and other medical problems.

Type of Information Offered

Health Resource is a medical information service that will provide the client with an individualized, in-depth research report on his or her specific health problem. The report will contain the latest information from medical texts and journals, as well as lay publications. The report will range from 110 to 150 pages and will list both traditional and alternative treatments. It will also inform the patient about research, new treatments, self-help measures, and physicians who specialize in the treatment of the specific disease. It will enable the patient to ask questions and participate in treatment decisions.

Costs

Comprehensive individualized report, $225 plus shipping. (Regular shipping: $4. Second-day air: $8. Overnight: $15.)

Method of Payment

Checks and money orders are accepted.

International Association of Cancer Victors and Friends

7740 West Manchester Avenue #110
Playa del Rey, California 90293
United States

(213) 822–5032

Primary Personnel

Ann Cinquina, editor of *Cancer Victors Journal*; Marie Steinmeyer, president.

Background

Founded in 1963 by Cecile Hoffman in San Diego, this association was created as an information organization specifically emphasizing nontoxic cancer therapies. An educational nonprofit corporation, the IACVF disseminates information concerning alternative cancer therapies. It reports on the most recent cancer studies and treatments. *Cancer Victors Journal* is published quarterly.

The following is a list of IACVF chapters and phone numbers. Contact international headquarters for exact addresses.

California
Playa del Rey: (213) 306–0748
Santa Barbara: (805) 969–9157
San Jose: (408) 269–7466
Salinas: (408) 663–5600

Florida
Fort Lauderdale: (305) 733–9121, 946–2770
Miami: (305) 271–2865
Orlando: (407) 859–1931
West Palm Beach: (407) 798–4536, 969–2810

Georgia
Atlanta: (404) 634–4101, 426–4399

Illinois
Cicero: (708) 780–6188
Niles: (708) 692–2596

Nevada
Las Vegas: (702) 795–4868

New Jersey
Matawan: (201) 583–1274

New York
Hicksville: (516) 796–3964

Texas
Amarillo: (806) 355–7782
El Paso: (915) 755–0724

Washington
Bothell: (206) 481–4351

Australia
Surrey Hills: 03–836–8764

Canada
Victoria: 478–8156

Illness Addressed

Cancer.

Type of Information Offered

Reports and information on alternative therapies and recent cancer studies.

Costs

Membership (yearly): $20.
Sustaining member: $100.
Life member: $250.
Perpetual member: $1,000.
Membership and donations are tax deductible.

International Health Information Institute

14417 Chase Street, Suite 432
Panorama City, California 91402
United States

Primary Personnel

Jack Tropp, director.

Background

Jack Tropp, a free-lance writer, lecturer, and consultant for more than 35 years, has been investigating and reporting on health and nutrition, with a sharp focus on holistic approaches to the treatment of cancer.

Jack Tropp was Japan correspondent for *Prevention Magazine*; research director of Shangri-La Natural Hygiene Institute, in Florida; director of Cancer Resource Center, in Los Angeles; and information and education director of Valley Cancer Institute, in Panorama City, California.

He received the Bronze Halo Award from the Southern California Motion Picture Council for his book *Cancer: A Healing Crisis—The Whole-Body Approach to Cancer Therapy*. The council cited the book as an "outstanding contribution to humanity."

Illness Addressed

Cancer.

Type of Information Offered

Jack can provide options, insights, and connections with physicians, holistic practitioners, clinics, and hospitals around the world to help sort the wheat from the chaff in today's imposing (ofttimes confusing) armamentarium of alternative/holistic modes, abundantly scattered over the landscape.

The institute does not diagnose, prescribe, or treat, but offers meaningful information and guidance—a blueprint, so to speak, to assist the inquirer with choices relative to the particular cancer problem. It is usually possible via first telephone contact to suggest a plan for follow-up.

Costs

Less than 30 minutes: $50.
At least 30 minutes but less than one hour: $75.
Also, there is a sliding scale, based on one's ability to pay. If additional research is necessary, then charges will be based on a case-by-case situation instead of on a straight time factor.

Method of Payment

Personal checks, traveler's checks, and money orders are accepted.

International Holistic Center Inc.

P.O. Box 15103
Phoenix, Arizona 85060
United States

(602) 957–3322

Contact Person

Stan Kalson, director.

Background

This organization provides information and referrals concerning holistic health care in Arizona and beyond.

Illness Addressed

Cancer and other diseases, plus a wellness approach to prevent illness.

Type of Information Offered

The center provides information about holistic health care and helps publish the *Holistic H.E.L.P. Handbook*. It offers massages, a support group, networking activities, information and referral services, and a speaker's bureau.

Related Readings

Holistic H.E.L.P. Handbook by Stan Kalson.

Holistic H.E.L.P. Directory.

Cassette tapes are also available. (Write to the center for a complete list.)

Costs

$10 for the handbook, $2 for the directory, and $6.95 for each cassette. Other costs not submitted for publication, but some of the services are free.

Medatic Research Inc.

1980 Coper Road
P.O. Box 360
Kelowna, British Columbia V1Y 6P7
Canada

(604) 862–3228

Primary Personnel

Leo Roy, B.A., M.D., N.D., F.A.N.A.

Background

Medatic Research is a computerized system for causal diagnosis and for the selection of possibly effective therapies. It is based on several ideas: that the only scientific and acceptable cure for cancer is the body's own immunity and resistance to the causes of disease; that the human body knows infinitely more about healing itself, even in conditions such as cancer, than science and all the healing professions ever will know; that clearly knowing the causes of any disease and understanding the effects each cause has on every biochemical and organ of the body is also to understand the therapies that need to be instituted; that prevention is the best cancer therapy; and that to measure the overall deviation from health is to measure proneness to cancer.

Illness Addressed

Cancer.

Type of Information Offered

Patients order a questionnaire, fill it in, and return it for computerized analysis. The computerized system searches out, tests, and evaluates each aspect of the patient's resistance and immunity; it correlates up to 25,000 bits of data to the causes of health breakdown (heredity, environment, stress, emotions, lifestyles and excesses, attitudes, personality complexes, deficiencies, toxicities, body structure, endocrinal and biochemical imbalances, life force reserves, etc.). It provides a printout, 12 to 15 pages, summarizing the patient's health problems. Patients submit the report to their holistic physician for correlation with the doctor's own findings and judgment and for individualizing therapies according to each patient's cancer. Medatic Research believes its system is most valuable when used in conjunction with other health-restoring programs, and it provides patients and doctors with consultants in the various fields of detoxification, nutrition, lifestyle, attitudes, and other health-restoring approaches.

Related Readings

Patient educational publications, audio cassettes, and videos are available. Send for complete list. (About 350 titles available.)

Costs

Questionnaire, mailings, and printout: $125.
Additional consultation (if required): $150.

National Health Federation

212 West Foothill Boulevard
P.O. Box 688
Monrovia, California 91016
United States

(818) 357–2181
(818) 359–8334

Primary Personnel

Maureen Salaman, president; Jay Arnoldus, chairman; Fred Nerio, executive director; Veronica A. Nerio, operations manager.

Background

National Health Federation is a non-profit consumer-oriented organization devoted exclusively to health matters. It is dedicated to preserving freedom of choice in health care issues—not only in the prevention of disease, but in the promotion of wellness.

There are approximately 80 active chapters around the country; for a listing, please write or call the Monrovia headquarters.

The federation has a full-time lobbyist, Richard Sellers, in Washington D.C. to defend health rights.

Illness Addressed

Cancer and other health problems.

Type of Information Offered

National Health Federation offers conventions, seminars, and a monthly news journal for members. Last year, conventions were held in Pasadena, California; Chicago (Rosemont), Illinois; San Francisco, California; Denver, Colorado; and Hollywood, Florida.

Costs

$36 for a regular membership ($24 for students and senior citizens over 65). $250 for life membership ($100 for students and senior citizens). $1,000 for perpetual membership.

National Self-Help Clearinghouse

25 West 43rd Street
Room 620
New York, New York 10036
United States

Primary Personnel

Frank Riessman, director; Audrey Gartner, executive director.

Background

The National Self-Help Clearinghouse was founded in 1976 to facilitate access to self-help groups and to increase awareness of the importance of mutual support groups. Self-help group members feel less isolated knowing others share similar problems; they exchange ideas and methods for handling problems; they actively work on their attitude and behavior to make positive changes in their lives; and they gain a sense of control over their own lives, leaving them less overwhelmed by their problems.

Illness Addressed

The whole range of life's crises.

Type of Information Offered

For a list of local self-help clearinghouses throughout the United States or for information about the location of a specific self-help group, just send in your inquiry along with a stamped, self-addressed envelope.

Costs

Publications are sold; inquiries are answered for free.
Self-Help Reporter, one-year subscription (four issues): $10.
How to Organize a Self-Help Group: $6.
Organizing a Self-Help Clearinghouse: $5.

Method of Payment

Personal checks are accepted.

Nutrition Education Association Inc.

3647 Glen Haven
Houston, Texas 77025
United States

P.O. Box 20301
Houston, Texas 77225
United States

(713) 665–2946

Primary Personnel

Ruth Yale Long, Ph.D., nutritionist.

Directions

Two miles west of medical center.

Background

Nutrition Education Association is a non-profit organization dedicated to educating the public about the importance of good nutrition for their health.

Illness Addressed

Cancer and various degenerative diseases.

Type of Information Offered

Nutrition education through books.

Related Readings

Crackdown on Cancer With Good Nutrition by Ruth Yale Long. Nutrition Education Association, 1983. Second edition 1989.

Home Study Course in the New Nutrition by Ruth Yale Long.

Switchover! The Anti-Cancer Cooking Plan for Today's Parents and Their Children by Ruth Yale Long.

These books are available through mail order.

Also recommended are books on nutrition by Jeffrey Bland, Linus Pauling, Roger Williams, and Emanuel Cheraskin.

Costs

Contact the Nutrition Education Association for a complete list of available books and their prices.

Patient Advocates for Advanced Cancer Treatments Inc. (PAACT)

1143 Parmelee N.W.
Grand Rapids, Michigan 49504
United States

(616) 453–1477
Fax: (616) 453–1846

Contact Person

Lloyd J. Ney, president; Gaylen Beverly, administrative assistant.

Background

PAACT claims to be the largest organization of its kind in the world, with more than 8,000 patients and more than 800 physicians of various disciplines counted among its members. PAACT's prostate cancer oncology group is a privately funded, cooperative research organization that investigates prostate cancer and its treatments.

Illness Addressed

Prostate cancer.

Type of Information Offered

State-of-the-art detection, diagnostics, evaluation, and treatments for all stages of prostate cancer and for related problems.

Related Readings

Onco-Logic (newsletter for physicians only).

Prostate Cancer Review.

Cancer Communication Newsletter.

"The Gland Illusion" in *American Health Magazine*. December 1990.

Costs

Voluntary donation and/or PAACT membership, which starts at $25.

Patient Rights Legal Action Fund

202 West 78th Street—3E
New York, New York 10024
United States

Primary Personnel

Avis Lang, coordinator.

Background

The Patient Rights Legal Action Fund was initially formed in August 1985 in response to what it deemed government violations of the basic constitutional rights of the cancer patients of Stanislaw R. Burzynski, M.D., Ph.D.

It organized a class action lawsuit to help ensure uninterrupted patient access to the clinic, stressing the return of past and present patients' medical records and insurance and billing files seized by the U.S. Food and Drug Administration in July 1985.

Although the patients' case was largely dismissed and the U.S. Supreme Court declined to hear an appeal of the dismissal, the case succeeded in becoming a focal point for educating the public about the problems of both doctors and patients who use nonstandard cancer therapies.

Related Readings

A booklet of excerpts from the 1,800-page official transcript of the October 1985 court hearing, including an introduction and explanatory notes. It is called *On The Public Record: Cancer Patients Take the U.S. Government to Court.*

A one-hour videotape, *Cancer Scandal: The Policies and Politics of Failure,* is also available. In the tape, three well-known science writers—Robert G. Houston, Patrick M. McGrady Jr., and Ralph W. Moss—explore the nature of the cancer industry in a no-holds-barred roundtable discussion.

Costs

The booklet costs $7.50, plus $1.50 postage and handling. The VHS videotape costs $29.95 plus $3 postage and handling. (Send a stamped, self-addressed envelope for additional articles and information.)

Method of Payment

Checks drawn on United States banks and postal money orders in United States dollars are accepted. Make payable to IFCO-PRLAF. All contributions are tax deductible.

People Against Cancer

P.O. Box 10
Otho, Iowa 50569–0010
United States

(515) 972–4444

Primary Personnel

Frank Wiewel, executive director and founder; Samuel S. Epstein, M.D., scientific director; and Ralph W. Moss, Ph.D., director of communications.

Background

People Against Cancer is a non-profit grassroots organization whose mission is to make deep inroads into the cancer problem by encouraging the development of innovative approaches and seeking new directions in the war on cancer. It works toward preserving, protecting, and enhancing medical freedom of choice. It promotes a pollution-free environment. Members include people with cancer, their loved ones, and others who are concerned with making rapid progress against the disease.

Illness Addressed

Cancer.

Type of Information Offered

People Against Cancer publishes and distributes books and other materials on innovative approaches to cancer prevention and treatment; it counsels members; it holds public and professional seminars; it addresses political issues; it provides information on the role of diet and nutrition in cancer; it helps people form self-help and empowerment groups; it teaches grassroots-organizing techniques; it arranges for members to receive discounts on medical-related travel costs; and it provides knowledgeable speakers on cancer for local groups, conventions, and the media.

Related Readings

Cancer Chronicles, a bimonthly newsletter.

Costs

Annual memberships cost $25 (regular), $50 (contributing), $100 (sustaining), and $200 (benefactor). The higher the level of membership, the more free books the member receives. Membership fee and donations are tax deductible.

Method of Payment

Checks, Visa, and MasterCard are accepted.

Planetree Health Resource Center

2040 Webster Street
San Francisco, California 94115
United States

(415) 923–3680

Primary Personnel

Tracey Cosgrove, M.L.I.S.

Background

Planetree is a non-profit consumer health library dedicated to helping patients and consumers become active participants in their own health and medical care. Planetree was founded in 1978 by a group of consumer advocates, educators, physicians, and business and cultural leaders.

Illness Addressed

Cancer and all medical conditions.

Type of Information Offered

A range of health and medical information—from lay-oriented publications to the latest professional literature to an extensive collection of alternative or complementary therapy books and journal articles.

   Planetree offers people who are unable to visit the library the following services:

Computer searched bibliography. Planetree will search the databases of the National Library of Medicine to produce a bibliography of up to 40 article citations. Citations include the available title, author, author address, source, and summaries of articles.

PDQ computer search. Sponsored by the National Cancer Institute, this database produces concise and current information on specific cancer diagnoses in a report format. Planetree provides both the "Information for Patients" and "State-of-the-Art Information" sections and details on prognosis, staging, and standard and investigational treatment protocols being conducted in the United States.

In-depth information packet. This is an individualized comprehensive selection of the current medical and lay literature on a diagnosis or topic, with particular emphasis on your focus of interest (e.g., complementary therapies). The packet is usually 50–60 pages and may include: selections from current medical textbooks, journals, and consumer health literature; materials describing complementary treatment options; a current computer search from medical literature databases; and the names and addresses of national and local organizations, support groups, or contact people dedicated to sharing information on your topic.

Costs

People who visit the library have access to all the information for free. People who cannot get to the library will be charged the following fees:
Computer searched bibliography: $25.
PDQ computer search: $25.
In-depth information packet: $75.

Method of Payment

Checks, money orders, cash, Visa, and MasterCard are accepted.

World Research Foundation

15300 Ventura Boulevard, Suite 405
Sherman Oaks, California 91403
United States

(818) 907–5483
Fax: (818) 907–6044

Contact Person

LaVerne Ross, vice president.

Primary Personnel

LaVerne Ross and Steven Ross, co-founders.

Background

Founded in 1984, World Research Foundation is a non-profit health and environmental information network. It includes five offices worldwide and an extensive library system containing books dating to the 1600s in English and 200 B.C. in other languages. The foundation is linked to more than 500 computer databases that provide access to important medical, scientific, and environmental information from more than 100 countries.

   The primary purpose of the organization is to locate, gather, codify, classify, and disseminate all available information dealing with health (both traditional and nontraditional, from ancient times to the present) and the environment. World Research Foundation's services are available to the public, health professionals, and the news media. The foundation acts as a consultant to governmental agencies. The foundation's research libraries are open to the public.

Illness Addressed

All diseases and illnesses.

Type of Information Offered

Two different types of health information files are available. A library search packet contains complementary, alternative, and nontraditional therapies gathered from books, periodicals, and other forms of literature. A computer search packet contains the most up-to-date allopathic (i.e., pharmaceutical and surgical) information, which tends to be very technical and uses medical terminology. The data is gathered from 5,000 medical journals worldwide and includes the latest 40–50 abstracted articles (when available).

Related Readings

World Research News, a quarterly newsletter, contains worldwide health information.

Also available are books, audio tapes and videotapes on numerous health topics.

Costs

Library search packet: $45 (California residents add sales tax).
Computer search packet: $45 (California residents add sales tax).
All donations are appreciated and tax deductible. For a $40 donation, you receive discounts on World Research Foundation health congresses, books, videotapes, and audio tapes, plus a subscription to the foundation's quarterly newsletter. For one dollar, you will receive a brochure on the foundation, a sample issue of *World Research News*, and a listing of available books, audio tapes, and videotapes.

Method of Payment

Visa, MasterCard, checks, and money orders are accepted.

Information Services

Overseas (Australia, United Kingdom)

Cancer Information & Support Society

39 Atchison Street
St. Leonard's
New South Wales 2065
Australia

(02) 906 2189

Other Branches

Gosford
(043) 28 4794

Hunter Valley
(049) 69 5566

Contact Person

Secretary.

Primary Personnel

Donald J. Benjamin.

Background

The society, a non-profit organization, was established in 1981 to provide people with information on holistic, nonaggressive, low-toxic methods that can help overcome disease.

Illness Addressed

Cancer and other degenerative diseases.

Type of Information Offered

Available in the office is a library, videos, tapes, research papers, information on overseas clinics, etc. Office hours are 10 a.m. to 4:30 p.m. Tuesday through Friday.

Related Readings

The society publishes a bimonthly newsletter and the *Cancer Information & Support Society Handbook.*

Costs

$25 for a one-year membership, which includes a subscription to the society's newsletter.

New Approaches to Cancer

5, Larksfield, Egham
Surrey, TW20 0RB
England
United Kingdom

(0784) 433610

Primary Personnel

Colin Ryder Richardson.

Background

New Approaches to Cancer, a registered charity, considers its holistic program to be a complement to the treatment of cancer as offered by the conventional medical profession. New Approaches acts as the nerve center of a network throughout the United Kingdom to promote research, organize workshops and conferences to improve attitudes, and show that cancer can be prevented and overcome.

It does not have its own clinic, but it does have 450 associates around the United Kingdom, ranging from individual therapists to support groups and residential clinics. It promotes the benefits of holistic and self-help methods of healing for those with cancer.

Illness Addressed

Cancer.

Type of Information Offered

Non-medical advice on the holistic approach to cancer.

Related Readings

The Holistic Approach to Cancer by Dr. Ian Pearce.

New Approaches to Cancer by Shirley Harrison.

The Bristol Programme by Penny Brohn.

Raw Energy by Leslie and Susannah Kenton.

How to Meditate by Dr. Lawrence LeShan.

Cancer as a Turning Point by Dr. Lawrence LeShan.

The Wealth Within by Dr. Ainslie Meares.

The Miracle of Colour Healing by Vicky Wall.

You Can Heal Your Life by Louise L. Hay. Coleman, 1985.

Emma Says Goodbye by Carolyn Nystrom.

Love, Medicine and Miracles by Dr. Bernie Siegel. Harper & Row, 1986.

Peace, Love and Healing by Dr. Bernie Siegel.

Getting Well Again by O. Carl Simonton, Stephanie Matthews-Simonton, and James Creighton. J.P. Tarcher, 1978.

Mind Over Cancer by Colin Ryder Richardson.

Costs

Costs not submitted for publication, but New Approaches to Cancer is a national registered charity.

Appendices

A Region-by-Region Look at Treatment Centers, Educational Centers, Support Groups, and Information Services

This region-by-region listing will help you locate those centers, services, and groups that can be found in your area. Each of these resources is discussed in detail in this book. The code letter following the entry will direct you to the section of the text containing complete information: **T** = Treatment Centers; **E** = Educational Centers; **S** = Support Groups; **I** = Information Services.

AUSTRALIA

(I.J.) Bullen **(E)**
Cancer Information & Support Society **(I)**
Cancer Support Association **(S)**
Gawler Foundation **(E)**
Hippocrates Health Centre of Australia **(E)**
International Association of Cancer Victors and Friends **(I)**
Meditation for Cancer Patients **(S)**
Nutrition & Stress Control Centre **(T)**
Radiant Health Centre **(E)**
Relaxation Centre of Queensland **(S)**

BAHAMAS

Immuno-Augmentative Therapy Centre **(T)**
Natural Health Center **(T)**

CANADA

Cancer Counselling Center **(S)**
Cancer Counselling Centre—Hope Program **(S)**
Cose **(T)**
Falk Oncology Centre **(T)**
International Association of Cancer Victors and Friends **(I)**
Medatic Research **(I)**
New Hope Naturopathic Medical Center **(T)**
Schafer's Health Centre **(T)**

ENGLAND

Bristol Cancer Help Centre **(T)**
Cheltenham Cancer Help Centre **(S)**
Chiltern Cancer Counselling **(S)**
Hereford Cancer Help Clinic **(S)**

LIFE Cancer Centre **(S)**
New Approaches to Cancer **(I)**
Newark Cancer Help Group **(S)**
Park Attwood Clinic **(T)**
Plymouth Natural Health and Healing
  Centre **(S)**
"Ray of Light" Spiritual Healing Centre
  (S)
St. Columba's House **(E)**
Thorpe Bay Self-Help Cancer Group **(S)**
Wessex Cancer Help Centre **(T)**

GERMANY

Chronic Disease Control and Treatment
  Center **(T)**
Gelsenkirken Immuno Therapy (GIT)
  Clinic **(T)**
Hufeland Klinik for Holistic
  Immunotherapy **(T)**
Institute for Immunology and Thymus
  Research **(T)**
(Robert) Janker Clinic **(T)**
Klinik Friedenweiler **(T)**
(Hans A.) Nieper, M.D. **(T)**
Veramed Klinik am Wendelstein **(T)**

GREECE

E.D. Danopoulos, M.D. **(T)**

JAPAN

Holistic Medical Clinic **(T)**
Institute for Religious Psychology **(S)**
Koda Clinic **(T)**
(Hotaka) Yojoen Holistic Health Center
  (E)

MEXICO

American Biologics—Mexico Medical
  Center **(T)**

American Metabolic Institute **(T)**
Bio-Medical Center **(T)**
Centro Medico Arturo Toledo **(T)**
(Yolanda) Fraire, M.D. **(T)**
Gerson Therapy—Hospital De Baja,
  California **(T)**
Hospital Ernesto Contreras **(T)**
Hospital Santa Monica **(T)**
Immune Therapy Clinic **(T)**
Instituto Cientifico de Regeneracion **(T)**
International Medical Center **(T)**
Manner Clinic **(T)**
Mission Medical Clinic **(T)**
Program for Studies of Alternative
  Medicines **(T)**
Sierra Clinic **(T)**

NETHERLANDS

Moerman Vereniging **(T)**

NEW ZEALAND

Bay of Plenty Chelation Clinic **(T)**
Herbal Education Resources Centre **(E)**
Medical Research **(E)**

PHILIPPINES

Manuel D. Navarro, M.D. **(T)**

SCOTLAND

Auchenkyle **(T)**

SPAIN

J. Buxalleu Font **(T)**

SWITZERLAND

Bircher-Benner Privatklinik **(T)**
Lukas Klinik **(T)**

UNITED STATES

North Central

(Brian E.) Briggs, M.D. **(T)**
Cancer Counseling Center of Ohio **(S)**
Cancer Treatment Centers of America **(T)**
Creative Health Institute **(E)**
(David P.) Goldberg, D.O., and Associates **(T)**
International Association of Cancer Victors and Friends **(I)**
Patient Advocates for Advanced Cancer Treatments **(I)**
People Against Cancer **(I)**
Shealy Institute for Comprehensive Health Care **(T)**
Waisbren Clinic **(T)**
Wellness Community **(S)**

Northeast

Atkins Center for Complementary Medicine **(T)**
(Seymour M.) Brenner, M.D. **(S)**
(Harold E.) Buttram, M.D. **(T)**
Center for Preventive Medicine and Dentistry **(T)**
Consciousness Research and Training Project **(S)**
Exceptional Cancer Patients **(S)**
Foundation for Advancement in Cancer Therapy **(I)**
(Nicholas) Gonzalez, M.D. **(T)**
Institute of Applied Biology **(T)**
International Association of Cancer Victors and Friends **(I)**
(P.) Jayalashmi, M.D. **(T)**

Kushi Institute **(E)**
(Lawrence) LeShan, Ph.D. **(S)**
Life-Affirming Support Group **(S)**
Mantell Medical Clinic **(T)**
National Self-Help Clearinghouse **(I)**
Patient Rights Legal Action Fund **(I)**
(Michael B.) Schachter, M.D., P.C., and Associates **(T)**
Syracuse Cancer Research Institute **(E)**
Wainwright House Cancer Support Program **(S)**
Wellness Community **(S)**
Wellspring Center for Life Enhancement **(S)**
(Ann) Wigmore Foundation **(E)**

South

Akbar Clinic **(T)**
(Paul) Beals, M.D. **(T)**
(Arlin J.) Brown Information Center **(I)**
Burzynski Research Institute **(T)**
Cancer Treatment Centers of America **(T)**
Center for Metabolic Disorders **(T)**
Center for Science in the Public Interest **(I)**
Gibson Clinic of Preventive Medicine **(T)**
Health Resource **(I)**
Hippocrates Health Institute **(E)**
Internal and Preventive Medical Clinic **(T)**
International Association of Cancer Victors and Friends **(I)**
Laboratory Atlanta **(T)**
Lost Horizon Health Awareness Center **(T)**
(Sandra) McLanahan, M.D. **(S)**
Nutrition Education Association **(I)**
Project Cure **(E)**
(Vladimir) Rizov, M.D. **(T)**
Ruscombe Mansion Community Health Center **(T)**
Southeast Research Foundation **(E)**
Warren's Clinic **(T)**

Wellness Community **(S)**

West

Alternative Health Center **(T)**
Biological Immunity Research Institute **(E)**
(Douglas) Brodie, M.D. **(T)**
(William M.) Buchholz, M.D., & Susan W.
  Buchholz, Ph.D. **(S)**
Cancer Control Society and Cancer Book
  House **(I)**
Cancer Federation **(I)**
Cancer Support Community **(S)**
Cancer Support and Education **(S)**
CanHelp **(I)**
Center for Attitudinal Healing **(S)**
Center for Cancer Survival **(S)**
Challenging Cancer **(S)**
Collaborative Medicine Center **(S)**
Colorado Outward Bound School **(S)**
Committee for Freedom of Choice in
  Medicine **(I)**
Commonweal Cancer Help Program **(S)**
GAM Diagnostic Nutritional Medical
  Center **(T)**
Healing Light Center Church **(S)**
Health Action **(E)**
Health Restoration Center **(T)**
Holistic Medical Center **(T)**
(Richard P.) Huemer, M.D. **(T)**
International Association of Cancer
  Victors and Friends **(I)**

International Association for Oxygen
  Therapy **(E)**
International Health Information Institute
  (I)
International Holistic Center **(I)**
Livingston Foundation Medical Center
  (T)
Los Angeles Healing Arts Center **(S)**
Meadowlark Health Center **(T)**
National Health Federation **(I)**
Nevada Clinic **(T)**
New Hope Institute **(S)**
Open Clinic **(T)**
Optimum Health Institute of San Diego
  (E)
(Linus) Pauling Institute of Science and
  Medicine **(E)**
Planetree Health Resource Center **(I)**
Private Cancer Clinic Tours **(S)**
(James R.) Privitera, M.D. **(T)**
Psychosomatics **(S)**
Simonton Cancer Center **(S)**
Tour of Cancer Clinics **(S)**
Valley Cancer Institute **(T)**
Vital-Life Institute **(T)**
Wellness Community **(S)**
Wellness Response Center **(S)**
World Research Foundation **(I)**

Puerto Rico

Ann Wigmore Research and Education
  Institute **(E)**

Glossary

Some of the terms that appear throughout this book may be unfamiliar to you. Although a number of these terms can be found in a standard medical dictionary, many are used strictly in the field of alternative therapy. This glossary defines those terms that are part of the vocabulary of alternative therapy—and even defines some terms that do not appear in this book. In addition, it defines many of the abbreviations that are used in these listings and in other literature on this subject.

Acupuncture is based on the theory that energy flows along specific pathways or "meridians" connecting the organs deep in the body with the acupoints on the surface of the body. In diseased conditions, there is a breakdown of the free flow of energy. By piercing the skin at certain points, the energy flow is stimulated or sedated so as to restore the functioning equilibrium.

AMID (Arthur morphologic immuno-status differential) is a microscopic examination of leukocytes (white blood cells) from specially prepared and stained thin blood films.

Amino acid therapy consists of infusions of protein to restore the body to a more natural condition. It is used in some metabolic cancer programs.

Amygdalin. *See* Laetrile.

Anabolic compounds allow the conversion of nutritive material into complex living matter in the constructive metabolism.

Anthroposophical medicine, developed by Rudolph Steiner, is a method of treating the whole body by addressing spiritual as well as physical aspects. Medications including mistletoe (*Viscum album*) as well as a special diet, color therapy, artistic therapy, curative eurythmy (movement), and specially prepared baths are included. It is widely available in special hospitals and clinics found mostly in Germany and Switzerland.

Antineoplastons, according to Dr. Stanislaw Burzynski, are a class of compounds produced by the living organism to protect it against neoplastic (tumorous) growth through a nonimmunological process that does not significantly inhibit the growth of normal tissue.

B.A. Bachelor of Arts.

B.Ac. Bachelor of Acupuncture.

Bach flower remedies are subtle essences originally refined in England. They are said to have powerful healing properties.

BCG (Bacillus Calmette-Guérin) is the tuberculosis vaccine that has been used in the treatment of cancer.

B.Ed. Bachelor of Education.

Beta-carotene is a derivative of vitamin A. It is widely accepted today as a cancer preventative.

Biofeedback is a technique based on the understanding that we can learn to regulate our own internal states, including that of the autonomic nervous system, which previously had been thought to be beyond our conscious control. Patients are hooked up to equipment that monitors their bodily functions and returns this information to the person in the form of visual, auditory, or tactile representations. It is said to be useful for controlling tension, migraine headaches, high blood pressure, anxiety, and insomnia. Through a series of sessions, the patient learns to trigger relaxation at will.

Biomagnetic and **micro frequencies**, according to some people, have the ability to destroy abnormal cells and harmful organisms, depending on the frequencies used.

Bovine cartilage is an immunostimulant used in treating cancer.

B.S. Bachelor of Science.

Butyrate complex is a combination of butyric acids. Its nontoxic fatty acids are used to stimulate interferon.

C.A. Certified Acupuncturist.

Catabolic actions break down complex compounds, taken as food, into simpler compounds.

CAT scan (computerized axial tomography scanning) involves the passing of numerous X-rays through the brain to produce a composite three-dimensional picture of it.

CBC (complete blood count) is a test that calculates the number of red and white cells per cubic millimeter of blood.

CEA (carcino-embryonic antigen) is a blood test used to determine the presence of cancerous cells.

Cell therapy, or cellular therapy, treats a diseased organ with the cells of a corresponding healthy organ. This consists of periodic injections of live or freeze-dried embryonic cells and tissues into the patient's muscular system. These injected cells are carried to the same type of cells within the body, where they work on the repair and revitalization of that tissue. Professor Niehans developed this method, which is popular in Europe. It is used to treat malignant diseases, diabetes, Down's syndrome, osteoporosis, central nervous system disorders, immune deficiency, impotence and sterility, and many other disorders. The embryonic cells used in the injections are usually removed from a healthy flock of black sheep.

Cesium chloride changes the pH of a cancer cell from acid to alkaline, making it difficult for the cell to reproduce and thereby slowing down growth, according to Dr. Keith Brewer. He says it does this without being toxic to normal cells.

Chelation therapy (EDTA): The word "chelation" is taken from the Greek "chele," which means to claw or pick up. The solution contains EDTA (ethylene diamine tetracetic acid), which carries out heavy metals like lead, cadmium, and arsenic, as well as other foreign substances, many of which enter our bodies in our food, in the air, and in our water. Chelation is the process of surrounding or enclosing a mineral atom with a larger protein molecule. The purpose is to increase the flow of blood to the vital organs and tissues of the body by reducing calcium deposits in the arteries and blood vessels.

Chemotherapy is the treatment of disease with chemical agents.

Chondroitin sulfate, pioneered in Germany, consists of mucopolysaturates that stimulate blood flow.

Clinical ecology is a relatively new branch of medicine focusing on environmentally provoked illnesses. These illnesses often seem to occur in man-made environments.

C.M.D. Doctor, Master in Surgery.

C.N. Clinical Nutritionist.

C.N.C. Certified Nutritional Consultant.

CoEnzyme Q-10 enhances body function by helping remove toxic foreign matter from the blood.

Coffee enemas are said to stimulate the liver to rid itself more effectively of deadly toxins. They were popularized in cancer treatment by Dr. Max Gerson and are used along with other cancer therapies as well. They must be prepared according to certain specifications.

Coley vaccine (toxins) incites a fever and is used in some cancer treatments.

Colonic irrigation is a gentle internal washing done by water under controlled pressure and temperature.

D.C. Doctor of Chiropractic.

D.D.S. Doctor of Dental Surgery.

D.H.M. Doctor of Homeopathic Medicine.

Diapulse treatment uses high-frequency electromagnetic energy to improve metabolism and general organ function.

D.M.D. Doctor of Dental Medicine.

DMSO (dimethyl sulfoxide) acts as an agent or vehicle that facilitates the penetration of anti-cancer drugs into the tumor.

D.N. Doctor of Naprapathy.

D.N.P. Doctor of Naturopathy.

D.O. Doctor of Osteopathy.

D.P. Doctor of Pharmacy.

D.P.M. Doctor of Podiatry.

D.Sc. Doctor of Science.

ECG (electrocardiogram) is a graphical record of cardiac function. The medical profession commonly refers to it as an EKG.

Ed.D. Doctor of Education.

EDTA. *See* Chelation therapy.

EKG. *See* ECG.

Essiac is an herbal concoction that has been widely used in Canada as a method of treating cancer. It is available through specific government approval of individual cases.

F.A.C.P. Fellow of the American College of Physicians.

F.C.A.P. Fellow of the College of American Pathologists.

Fever therapy, or pyretotherapy, has been found to be beneficial to the body in that lymphocytes will produce a great amount of antibodies when the body's temperature is high. These antibodies will destroy bacteria and toxins and help eliminate them, thus stimulating the immune system to work against the cancer. Fever is induced through the injection of a bacterial substance into the body.

Flutamide gets positive results with prostate cancer, according to discoveries by Dr. LaBrie in Canada.

Fred (fiche reticular endithelial differential) tests were developed by Dr. Yves Augusti of France for determining the presence of cancer.

Germanium, a natural substance found in plants and foods, was found in Japan to be an oxygen enhancer, restoring to normal function the T-cells, the B-lymphocytes natural killer cell activity, and numbers of antibody-forming cells.

GH3, or Gerovital H3, was developed in Romania by Ana Aslan, M.D. It is used to treat a variety of degenerative conditions and to slow the aging process.

Hair analysis is painless, easy, and free of risks. A small amount of hair is taken from the nape of the neck to examine the intracellular (inside the cell) information of the person's condition for the last three months. This procedure reveals toxic metal levels and nutrient mineral levels.

H.D. Homeopathic Doctor.

Herbal therapy uses various herbal combinations for healing as well as cleansing purposes. These are used in the form of tablets, capsules, tinctures, extracts, and herbal baths with poultices. Herbs are a valuable adjunct to many therapies.

HLB (Hyton-Lygard Bradford) blood tests are used on patients to monitor the progress of their disease.

H.M.D. Holistic Medical Doctor; Homeopathic Doctor.

Homeopathy is a system of medicine based on the belief that the cure of disease can be effected by minute doses of substances that, if given to a healthy person in large doses, would produce the same symptoms as are present in the disease being treated. Homeopathy employs natural substances in small doses to stimulate the body's reactive process to remove toxic waste and bring the body back into balance. It was first used in the early 1800s by Samuel Hahnemann of Germany.

Hydrazine sulfate is an inexpensive chemical substance used to treat cachexia (wasting away). It is said to have anti-cancer properties.

Hydrogen peroxide, properly prepared and given orally or by infusion, is used to increase oxygen tension in the cancer cell. It is used for other degenerative diseases, too.

Hydrotherapy can include steam baths, whirlpools, foot baths, and mineral baths, all of which help remove toxins from the body, stimulate the entire nervous and muscular system, and increase circulation.

Hyperthermia is the artificial induction of exceptionally high fever for therapeutic purposes. Malignant cells cannot tolerate heat as well as normal cells can; therefore, the increased temperature destroys cancer cells and leaves normal cells intact. There are several ways of using hyperthermia, ranging from wet heat to dry heat.

Immunology is the science dealing with the specific mechanisms by which living tissues react to foreign biological material in a way that may enhance resistance or immunity. In mainstream medicine, such treatments include the use of monoclonal antibodies, interferon, interleukin-2, and TNF (tumor necrosis factor).

Immunotherapies are those therapies that strengthen the immune system. There is a wide range of therapies that are said to operate this way.

Interferon is a protein molecule that is created by white blood cells. It acts to keep viruses from multiplying.

Interleukins are hormone-like substances produced by lymphocytes. They often are used in mainstream biological therapies having strong side effects.

Iridology is the science of determining acute, sub-acute, chronic, and destructive stages in the affected organs of the body by examining their corresponding areas in the iris.

Iscador, or mistletoe, is an herb used mainly as an anti-cancer agent in anthroposophical medicine.

Jason Winters herbal tea is a combination of three herbs—red clover, chapperal, and an Oriental herb—that cured Jason Winters of his cancer.

Kirlian photography is a method of photographing objects by means of high-voltage spark discharges. The Kirlians describe their photography as a method for the conversion of properties of an object into electrical properties that are then captured on film.

Koch reagent (glyoxilide) is an oxidation catalyst used in very low dosage. It is believed to stimulate biochemical reactions that antagonize malignant cells. It is usually administered by injection into the muscle. The theory is that the anaerobic (non-oxidizing) metabolism of malignant cells may be part of the cause of malignancy, as well as an identifying characteristic of cancer cells. Stimulating oxidation results in an environment less favorable to cancer cells.

Laetrile (amygdalin) has been used as an anti-cancer agent. Although it is not a vitamin, this substance is also known as vitamin B_{17}. Drs. Ernest Krebs Jr. and Sr. did research with amygdalin. They found that it helped relieve pain and increase appetite, weight, and energy. Laetrile is used as a part of metabolic therapy that includes a special laetrile diet, and as part of an enzyme therapy that helps open the outer coat of the cancer cell. Then the cyanide in the laetrile and the body's own immune system are said to destroy the cancer cell. Benzaldahyde, another component, has been found to help in relieving pain.

M.A. Master of Arts.

M.Ac. Master of Acupuncture.

Macrobiotics is a lifestyle and diet adapted from the Far East and made known in America by Michio Kushi. The principles of the diet consist of balancing the yin and yang energies of foods. In brief, yin foods, such as water, are expansive, while yang foods, such as salt or meat, are constrictive. For the most part, the diet consists of whole grain cereals, millet, rice, soups, and vegetable dishes, with beans and supplementary foods depending on the individual and the condition. Different types of cancers are considered either yin or yang, and the macrobiotic program must be adapted to each individual.

M.D. Doctor of Medicine.

Metabolic therapy usually consists of daily doses of amygdalin (laetrile), enzymes, and vitamin-mineral supplements. A diet is often recommended to complement this program. The diet centers on avoiding fats, salts, and sugars, and on eating plenty of raw vegetables and fruits.

M.H. Master Herbalist.

Monoclonal antibodies attack tumor antigens in specific cancers and are part of mainstream immunotherapy.

M.S. Master of Science.

M.Sc.D. Doctor of Medical Science.

M.S.N. Master of Science in Nursing.

M.S.W. Master of Social Work.

Naturopathy is a natural way to heal using many methods, including herbs, diet, osteopathy, hydrotherapy, sunlight, deep breathing, exercise, relaxation, and the removal of noxious influences.

N.D. Doctor of Naturopathy.

Noninvasive vascular testing is an electronic analysis of circulation. Changes in blood vessel walls in smokers and in patients suffering from diabetes, arteriosclerosis, and other causes of circulatory problems can be detected and analyzed.

Nuclear medicine is the branch of medicine that deals with the use of radioisotopes in diagnosis and therapy.

O.D. Doctor of Optometry.

O.M.D. Oriental Medicine Doctor.

Osteopathy is a school of healing that teaches that the body is a vital mechanical organism whose structural and functional integrity are coordinated and interdependent and that the abnormality of either constitutes disease. Its major contribution to treatment is manipulation.

Ozone: Medical ozone is made by causing medically pure oxygen to flow over electrically charged surfaces. It is used mainly in three ways. One is to flow ozone gas over open lesions such as diabetic gangrene on feet, hands, arms, or legs. The ozone often eliminates any need for amputation of the extremity by destroying infections and promoting normal healing. Intravenous injections of ozone directly into the blood stream is another means of using ozone. The tiny bubbles formed when the ozone-oxygen is slowly injected through a fine needle are quickly dissolved into the blood stream. The third way is for ozone-oxygen to be introduced into the colon of adults. Ozone may help to destroy parasites and bacteria throughout the colon.

PABA (p-aminobenzoic acid) is a protective antioxidant vitamin used by the skin to filter out damaging ultraviolet radiation.

Pao D'Arco Herbal Tea, or lapochol or taheebo, is a South American tea made from tree bark generally found in Brazil or Argentina. The tea is said to have anti-cancer properties.

P.D. Doctor of Pharmacy.

Phar.G. Graduate in Pharmacy.

Phar.M. Master of Pharmacy.

Ph.C. Pharmaceutical Chemist.

Ph.D. Doctor of Philosophy.

Ph.T. Physical Therapist.

Plasmapheresis is employed as a therapeutic procedure in the treatment of several diseases. This procedure separates blood into its various components, isolating the plasma, red cells, white cells, and platelets in a continuous flow system. The typical plasmapheresis procedure involves separating the patient's red blood cells from the plasma. The red blood cells are then immediately returned to the patient, and the volume of plasma removed is replaced with fresh frozen plasma or with normal saline solution and albumin, which have properties similar to plasma. Plasmapheresis can also be used on some cancer patients, such as those whose tumors produce high quantities of abnormal proteins (e.g., multiple myeloma and related disorders). The plasmapheresis separates these proteins by removing the patient's plasma and replacing it with other compatible solutions.

P.M.D. Private Medical Doctor.

Polypeptides are compounds containing two or more amino acids united through the linkage of peptides, intermediates between the amino acids, and peptones in the synthesis of proteins.

Progenator cryptocides is a microbe, or bacterium, that is in the blood and can be seen through a darkfield microscope. According to Dr. Virginia Livingston, this microbe is the cause of cancer.

Proteolytic enzymes have a particular ability to break down certain proteins yet do not attack the beneficial proteins that make up the normal cells of the body. These enzymes are said to have great value in fighting cancer as well as many other diseases. If the body were always capable of producing adequate proteolytic enzymes, it is possible that cancer would not develop. In theory, cancer cells have a type of protein coating that is destroyed by proteolytic enzymes. When this protein is destroyed, the body's white cells are able to attack the cancer cells and destroy them.

Psychic surgery is performed most frequently in the Philippines by psychic healers, who use only their hands to "remove" impurities from the patient's body. Reputedly, this surgery is quick and relatively painless. The healer closes up the "incision," no scar remains, and it takes very little time.

P.T. Physical Therapist.

Qi Gung, a Chinese form of yoga, is said to be very helpful in treating cancer. Its efficacy in the treatment of lung cancer is under investigation.

Radiation therapy is usually treatment with ionizing radiation, including Roentgen rays, radium, or other radioactive substances.

R.C.P. Respiratory Care Practitioner.

Rife microscope, developed by Dr. Royal Rife, enabled him to see harmful cells destroyed.

R.N. Registered Nurse.

Rolfing is a form of deep muscle body work developed by the late Dr. Ida Rolf.

R.P.T. Registered Physical Therapist.

714X is a camphor-based nontoxic substance that works against cancer, according to observations through a powerful microscope known as a Somatoscope. Gaston Naessens created both 714X and the Somatoscope.

Shark cartilage is an anti-cancer immunostimulant.

Shark liver extract, researched in Sweden as being helpful in leukemia cases, is now being used with other cancers, too.

Staphage-lysate is a microbial accumulation used to stimulate an immune response. It is sometimes called "the germ's germ."

Visualization is the use of mental imagery to create positive beliefs that will activate the body's defenses against disease. In visualization, images are perceived in the mind with such distinctness that they seem to be seen by the eyes.

Yoga (from the Sanskrit word for "union" or "oneness") is a personal self-help system of health care and spiritual development. Its founders were working in India about 2,000 years ago. This approach to becoming one with life involves meditation; postures or asanas, known as Hatha yoga; service to others, known as Karma yoga; devotion and love, known as Bhakti yoga; a vegetarian diet; and breathing methods that help calm the body and mind.

Bibliography

Because a great deal of literature has been written about the world of alternatives in the field of cancer, the following list has been divided into four categories to help you find those books that are of greatest interest to you. Many, but not all, duplicate the Related Readings listed in the text. By no means does this bibliography include all of the books that have been written on this subject over the years.

Specific regimens can be found under "Program-Related Books." As far as possible, the regimen has been indicated whenever the title isn't self-explanatory. The "Survivor Stories" category includes firsthand accounts of patients' recoveries. In most cases, the therapy used has been indicated. Under "Mind: Behavioral-Psychological Aspects of Health," you will find many of the more important books in this growing area. "General Reading" is a kind of catchall for books that sometimes touch on one or more of the above subjects, and sometimes encompass much more. Additional regimens and programs, as well as books on the politics of cancer, can be found here.

If a book is not available through conventional sources and is still in print, try a center that is related to the subject matter, or contact the

Cancer Book House
2043 North Berendo Street
Los Angeles, California 90027

PROGRAM-RELATED BOOKS

Amygdalin (Laetrile) Therapy. Bruce W. Halstead, M.D. Choice Publications, Inc., 1977.

An Anthroposophical Approach to Cancer. Rita Leroi, M.D. Mercury Press, 1982.

Be Your Own Doctor: A Positive Guide to Natural Living. Ann Wigmore. Avery Publishing Group, 1982. (Wheatgrass and Raw Foods)

Biologically Closed Electric Circuits. Bjorn E.W. Nordenstrom. Stockholm: Nordic Medical Publications, 1983. (Altering Electrical Fields)

Bristol Programme. Penny Brohn. Century Hutchinson, 1987.

Cancer: A Mandate to Humanity. Friedrich Lorenz. Mercury Press, Fellowship Community, 1982. (Anthroposophical Medicine)

Cancer: A New Breakthrough. Virginia Livingston-Wheeler, M.D. Livingston, 1972. (Livingston Treatment)

Cancer: A Second Opinion. Josef Issels, M.D. London: Hodder and Stoughton, 1975. (Issels Treatment)

Cancer and the Philosophy of the Far East. George Ohsawa. George Ohsawa Macrobiotic Foundation, 1981. (Macrobiotic Diet)

Cancer: Causes, Prevention and Treatment: The Total Approach. Paavo Airola. Health Plus Publishers, 1982. (Metabolic)

Cancer Holiday. Bettie Towner. Greenlake Publishers, 1978. (Discusses Several Clinics)

The Cancer Prevention Diet. Edward Esko, Editor. East West Foundation, 1981. (Macrobiotic Diet)

The Cancer Prevention Diet. Michio Kushi and Alex Jack. St. Martin's Press, 1983. (Macrobiotic Diet)

The Cancer Problem. Paul Niehans. Staempfli & Cie Ltd., 1969. (Cell Therapy)

Cancer Prophylaxis and Cancer Immunology. Paul Niehans. Staempfli & Cie Ltd., 1968. (Cell Therapy)

A Cancer Therapy: Results of 50 Cases. Max Gerson, M.D. Totality Books, 1977. (Gerson Therapy)

Cleanse. Jason Winters. Vinton Publishing, 1984. (Jason Winters Program)

The Conquest of Cancer: Transcript From a Videotape Program. Virginia Livingston-Wheeler, M.D., and Owen Wheeler, M.D. (Livingston Treatment)

The Conquest of Cancer: Vaccines and Diet. Virginia Livingston-Wheeler, M.D., with Edmond G. Addeo. Franklin Watts Publishing, 1984. (Livingston Treatment)

The Death of Cancer. Harold W. Manner. Advanced Century Publishing, 1978. (Manner Metabolic Protocol)

Diagnosis: Cancer—Prognosis: Life (the Story of Dr. Lawrence Burton). Jane Riddle Wright. Albright and Co., 1985. (Burton's Immuno-Augmentative Therapy)

Diet for Cancer. Virginia Livingston, M.D. (Livingston Treatment)

Dr. Kelley's Answer to Cancer. (Combines *One Answer to Cancer* by Kelley with *Metabolic Ecology* by Rohe.) Wedgestone Press, 1986.

Dr. Moerman's Anti-Cancer Diet. Ruth Jochems. Avery Publishing Group, 1990.

Dr. Nieper's Revolution. Hans Nieper, M.D. (Nieper Program)

An End to Cancer. Leon Chaitow, D.O. Wellingsborough, Northamptonshire, England: Thorens Publishers Ltd., 1985. (Dr. Chaitow's Program)

The Famous Bristol Detox Diet. Alec Forbes, M.D. Keats Publishing, Inc. (Bristol Cancer Help Centre)

Galileo of the Microscope. Christopher Bird. Les Presses de l'Université de la Personne Inc., 1990. (Gaston Naessens)

A Gentle Way With Cancer. Brenda Kidman. London: Century Publishing, 1985. (Bristol Cancer Help Centre)

Gerson Therapy Handbook. Mary Lee Rork. 1981.

The Grape Cure. Johanna Brandt. Ehret Literature Publishing Co.

Homeopathic Medicine and Cancer. Robin Murphy. Homeopathic Research Project, National College of Naturopathic Medicine, 1979.

International Protocols IIMP in Cancer Management. Robert W. Bradford et al. Robert W. Bradford Foundation, 1982. (American Biologics)

Killing Cancer: The Jason Winters Story. Jason Winters. England: Skilton and Shaw Publishing, 1980. (Jason Winters Herbal Tea)

Koch Remedy/Cancer. Borderland Sciences Research Foundation, 1986.

Laetrile: Case Histories. John A. Richardson, M.D., and Patricia Griffin. Bantam, 1977.

Laetrile/Control for Cancer. Glenn D. Kittler. Warner Paperback, 1973.

Little Cyanide Cookbook—B17 Recipes. June de Spain. American Media, 1978. (Laetrile Therapy)

The Macrobiotic Approach to Cancer. Michio Kushi. Avery Publishing Group, 1982.

The Macrobiotic Cancer Prevention Cookbook. Aveline Kushi with Wendy Esko. Avery Publishing Group, 1988.

A Matter of Life or Death: The Incredible Story of Krebiozen. Herbert Bailey. G.P. Putnam's Sons, 1958. (Krebiozen and Dr. Andrew Ivy)

Metabolic Cancer Therapies. Kurt W. Donsbach, M.D. International Institute of Natural Health Sciences, Inc., 1981.

Metabolic Cancer Therapy. Bruce W. Halstead, M.D. Golden Quill Publishers, Inc., 1978.

Metabolic Ecology: A Way to Win the Cancer War. Fred Rohe. Wedgestone Press, 1982. (Kelley Treatment)

The Metabolic Management of Cancer. Robert W. Bradford and Michael L. Culbert, Editors. Robert W. Bradford Foundation, 1979. (American Biologics)

Metabolic Therapy, A-1982 and C-1982. Dr. Harold W. Manner. Metabolic Research Foundation. (Manner Protocol)

The Microbiology of Cancer. Virginia Livingston-Wheeler, M.D. (Livingston Treatment)

The New Approach to Cancer. Cameron Stauth. English Brothers Press, 1982. (Kelley Treatment)

New Hope for Cancer Victims. William Donald Kelley, D.D.S. The Kelley Research Foundation, 1980. (Kelley Treatment)

Nutrition: The Cancer Answer. Maureen Salaman. Statford Publishing, 1983.

One Answer to Cancer. William Donald Kelley, D.D.S. Wedgestone Press, Kelley Research Foundation, 1974. (Kelley Treatment)

Raw Food Treatment Cancer/Other. Kristine Nolfi, M.D. Health Research.

Rejuvenation. Stephen Blauer. Green Gown Publications. (Raw Foods)

Research in Physiopathology as Basis of Guided Chemotherapy With Special Application to Cancer. Emanuel Revici, M.D. Van Nostrand, 1961. (Revici Treatments)

Revolution in Technology, Medicine and Society. Hans Nieper, M.D. Oldenburg: MIT Verlag, 1983. (Nieper)

Second Opinion: LaPacho and the Cancer Controversy. Bill Wead. Canada: Rostrom, 1985. (Pao D'Arco Herbal Tea)

Survival Into the 21st Century. Viktoras Kulvinskas. Omangod Press, 1975. (Wheatgrass and Raw Foods)

The Treatment of Cancer With Herbs. John Heinerman. BiWorld Publishers, 1980.

The Truth About Perisel. Jason Winters. M & R Publishers, 1982. (Jason Winters)

Why Suffer? Ann Wigmore. Avery Publishing Group, 1985. (Wheatgrass and Raw Foods)

The Yeast Connection. William Crook, M.D. Professional Books, 1986. (Anti-Candida)

You Don't Have to Die. Harry M. Hoxsey. Joseph C. Carl, 1977. (Hoxsey)

SURVIVOR STORIES

Cancer—One Man's Fight to Control Malignancy. Robert Stickle. Natural Foods Associates, 1976.

Cancer Winner. Jaquie Davison. Pacific Press, 1977. (Gerson)

Confessions of a Kamikaze Cowboy. Dirk Benedict. Avery Publishing Group, 1991. (Macrobiotics)

Gentle Giants. Penny Brohn. London: Century Publishing. (Issels)

How I Conquered Cancer Naturally. Eydie Mae Hunsberger. Harvest House, 1975. (Wheatgrass and Raw Foods)

How I Healed My Cancer Holistically. Dore Deverell. Psychenutrition, Inc., 1978. (Kelley Treatment)

How I Overcame Inoperable Cancer. Wong Hon Sung. Exposition Press, 1975.

I Beat Cancer. Bernice Wallin. Contemporary Books, 1978. (BCG Vaccine)

I Fought Leukemia and Won. Rex B. Eyre. Hawkes Publishing, 1982. (Gerson)

My God, I Thought You'd Died. Claude Dosdall and Joanne Broatch. Bantam-Seal Books, 1986.

My Triumph Over Cancer. Beata Bishop. Keats Publishing, Inc., 1986. (Gerson)

A Rational Concept of Cancer. Robert Stickle. Natural Foods Associates, 1977.

Recalled by Life. Anthony Sattilaro, M.D. Avon Books, 1982. (Macrobiotics)

Thank God I Had Cancer. Rev. Clifford Oden. Cancer Book House, 1984.

Too Young to Die. Rick Hill. Hill Publications, 1979. (Contreras)

Vital Signs. Fitzhugh Mullan, M.D. Dell Publishing Co., Inc., 1983.

You Bet You Can. Tony Moscato, 1984. (Jason Winters Tea/Wheatgrass)

You Can Conquer Cancer. Ian Gawler. Australia: Hill of Content Publishing, 1985. (Gerson, Megavitamins, Psychic Surgery, Meditation)

MIND: BEHAVIORAL-PSYCHOLOGICAL ASPECTS OF HEALTH

Bridges of the Bodymind. Jeanne Achterberg and G. Frank Lawlis. Institute for Personality and Ability Testing, 1980.

Cancer as a Turning Point. Lawrence LeShan. Plume, 1990.

From Victim to Victor. Harold Benjamin, Ph.D. Dell, 1987.

Getting Well Again. O. Carl Simonton, M.D., Stephanie Matthews-Simonton, and James Creighton. J.P. Tarcher, 1978.

The Healing Family. Stephanie Matthews-Simonton. Bantam Books, 1984.

The Healing Mind. Irving Oyle. Celestial Arts, 1979.

Healing With Mind Power. Richard Shames, M.D. Rodale Press, 1978.

Healing With the Mind's Eye. Michael Samuels, M.D., with Nancy Samuels. Summitt, 1990.

The Human Patient. Naomi Remen, M.D. Anchor Press/Doubleday, 1980.

Hypnosis and Behavioral Medicine. Daniel P. Brown and Erika Fromm. Lawrence Erlbaum Associates Publishing, 1987.

Imagery in Healing: Shamanism and Modern Medicine. Jeanne Achterberg. Shambhala Publications, 1985.

Imagery of Cancer. Jeanne Achterberg and G. Frank Lawlis. Institute for Personality and Ability Testing, 1978.

Love Is Letting Go of Fear. Gerald G. Jampolsky, M.D. Celestial Arts, 1979.

Love, Medicine, and Miracles. Bernie S. Siegel, M.D. Harper & Row Publishers, 1986.

Mind and Immunity: Behavioral Immunology. Steven E. Locke and Mady Hornig-Rohan. Institute for the Advancement of Health.

Mind Over Cancer. Colin Ryder Richardson. Great Britain: W. Foulsham & Co., 1988.

Minding the Body, Mending the Mind. Joan Borysenko. Bantam New Age Books, 1988.

Peace, Love, and Healing. Bernie S. Siegel, M.D. Harper & Row, 1989.

The Psychobiology of Mind-Body Healing. Ernest Lawrence Rossi. W.W. Norton & Co., Inc., 1986.

Psychological and Behavioral Treatments for Disorders Associated With the Immune System: An Annotated Bibliography. Steven E. Locke. Institute for the Advancement of Health.

Superimmunity. Paul Pearsall, Ph.D. Fawcett, 1987.

You Can Fight for Your Life. Lawrence LeShan. M. Evans and Co., 1977.

You Can Heal Your Life. Louise Hay. Coleman, 1985.

GENERAL READING

AIDS, Cancer and the Medical Establishment. Raymond Keith Brown, M.D. Robert Speller Publishers, 1986.

Anatomy of an Illness. Norman Cousins. W.W. Norton and Co., 1979.

The Beneficial Effects of Bacterial Infections on Host Resistance to Cancer: End Results in 449 Cases. Helen Coley Nauts. Cancer Research Institute, Inc.

Beneficial Effects of Immunotherapy on Sarcoma of the Soft Tissues, Other Than Lymphosarcoma. Helen Coley Nauts. Cancer Research Institute, Inc.

Breast Cancer: A Nutritional Approach. Carlton Fredericks. Grosset & Dunlap, 1977.

Breast Cancer: Immunological Factors Affecting Incidence, Prognosis and Survival. Helen Coley Nauts. Cancer Research Institute, Inc.

Cancer: A Healing Crisis. Jack Tropp. Exposition Press, 1980. (Gerson/Issels)

Cancer and Consciousness. Barry Bryant. Sigo Press, 1990.

Cancer and Its Nutritional Therapies. Richard Passwater. Keats Publishing, Inc., 1983.

Cancer and Vitamin C. Ewan Cameron and Linus Pauling. Linus Pauling Institute of Science and Medicine, 1979.

The Cancer Biopathy. Wilhelm Reich. Farrar, Straus, and Giroux, 1973.

The Cancer Blackout. Maurice Natenberg. Cancer Book House, 1975.

The Cancer Blackout Amended. Nat Morris. Regent House, 1976.

Cancer Causes and Natural Controls. Lynn Dallin. Ashley Books, 1983.

The Cancer Connection. Larry Agran. St. Martin's Press, 1977.

The Cancer Conspiracy. Dr. Robert E. Netterberg and Robert T. Tailor. Pinnacle Books, 1981.

The Cancer Cure That Worked. Barry Lynes. Canada: Marcus Books, 1987.

Cancer, Disease of Civilization. Ebba Waerland. Provoker Press, 1980.

The Cancer Industry: Unraveling the Politics. Ralph W. Moss. Paragon House, 1989.

Cancer, Metabolic Therapy and Laetrile. Douglas Heinsohn, 1977.

Cancer: Myths and Realities of Cause and Cure. M.L. Kothari and L.A. Mehta. Marion Boyars, Inc., 1979.

Cancer 1985. Hellfried Sartori, M.D. Life Science Universal, 1984.

A Cancer Patient's Survival Manual. Barbara Huntington. Avant Publishing, 1983.

Cancer Prevention, Fallacies and Some Reassuring Facts. Cyril Scott. England: Athene Publishing Co., Ltd., 1968.

The Cancer Survivors and How They Did It. Judith Glassman. Dial Press, 1983.

The Cancer Syndrome. Ralph W. Moss. Grove Press, 1980.

Cancer? Think Curable! The Gerson Therapy. S.J. Haught. Gerson Institute, 1983.

Cancer Treatment: Why So Many Failures? Richard Ericson. GE-PS Cancer Memorial, 1980.

Confessions of a Medical Heretic. Robert Mendelsohn. Warner Books, 1980.

Coronary? Cancer? God's Answer: Prevent It! Richard Brennan. Harvest House, 1979.

Crackdown on Cancer With Good Nutrition. Ruth Yale Long. Nutrition Education Association, 1983.

Diet, Nutrition, and Cancer. Committee on Diet, Nutrition, and Cancer, Assembly of Life Sciences, National Research Council. National Academy Press, 1982.

Divided Legacy—A History of the Schism in Medical Thought (3 Vols.). Harris Livermore Coulter. North Atlantic Books, 1982.

Dr. Atkins' Health Revolution: How Complementary Medicine Can Extend Your Life. Bantam, 1990.

Food Is Your Best Medicine. Henry G. Bieler, M.D. Vintage Books, 1973.

Food Pharmacy. Jean Carper. Bantam, 1988.

Foods that Heal. Maureen Salaman. Statford Press, 1989.

Foods that Heal. Dr. Bernard Jensen. Avery Publishing Group, 1988.

Formula For Life. Eberhard Kronhausen, Ed.D., and Phyllis Kronhausen, Ed.D., with Harry B. Demopoulos, M.D. 1989.

Free Radical—Albert St. Gyorgyi and the Battle Over Vitamin C. Ralph W. Moss. Paragon House, 1988.

Freedom From Cancer. Mike Culbert. 76 Press, 1976.

The Great Medical Monopoly Wars. P.J. Lisa. International Health Institute of Natural Health Sciences, 1986.

Green Barley Essence. Yoshihide Hagiwara, M.D. Keats Publishing, 1986.

The Healing of Cancer. Barry Lynes. Marcus Books, 1989.

Health and Healing. Andrew Weil, M.D. Houghton Mifflin Co., 1983.

Health Through God's Pharmacy. Maria Treben. Austria: Wilhelm Ennsthaler, 1984.

How to Prevent and Gain Remission From Cancer. John Tobe. Canada: Provoker Press, 1975.

The Indispensable Cancer Handbook. Kathryn H. Salsbury and Eleanor Liebman Johnson. Wideview Books/PEI Books, Inc., 1981.

Integral Cancer Therapies. Michael Lerner. Commonweal, 1987.

Maria Treben's Cures. Maria Treben. Austria: Wilhelm Ennsthaler, 1986.

Meals That Heal. L. Anne Fransen. Nutritional Research and Development, 1985.

Medical Dark Ages Circa 1984 or Cancer Alternative Therapies Cure Rates. Ralph Hovnanian. 1984.

Medical Nemesis. Ivan Illich. Bantam Books, 1976.

Medicine on Trial. Charles B. Inlander, Lowell S. Levin, and Ed Weiner. People's Medical Society, 1988.

Miracle Cure: Organic Germanium. Kazuhiko Asai, M.D. Harper & Row, 1987.

Natural Health, Natural Medicine. Andrew Weil, M.D. Houghton Mifflin, 1990.

New Hope and Improved Treatments for Cancer Patients. David Holmes. England: Wentworth House.

New Hope for Cancer Victims. Richard Welch, M.D. Cancer Book House, 1965.

No More Cancer. Ruth Yale Long. Nutrition Education Association, Inc.

Now That You Have Cancer. Robert W. Bradford. Choice Publication, 1977. (American Biologics)

Osteogenic Sarcoma: End Results Following Immunotherapy with Bacterial Vaccines: 165 Cases or Following Bacterial Infections Inflammation or Fever: 41 Cases. Helen C. Nauts. Cancer Research Institute, Inc.

The Politics of Cancer. Samuel S. Epstein, M.D. Anchor Press, Doubleday, 1979.

Prevention and Cure of Cancer. Mulhim A. Hassan, M.D. Exposition Press, 1983. (Focal Infection)

The Prime Cause and Prevention of Cancer. Otto Warburg. Cancer Book House, 1973.

Repression and Reform in the Evaluation of Alternative Cancer Therapies. Robert G. Houston. IAT Patients' Association, 1988.

Survival Factor in Neoplastic and Viral Diseases. William Koch, M.D. Cancer Book House.

The Stress of Life. Hans Selye, M.D. McGraw-Hill Book Co., 1978.

Tijuana Clinics—Questions and Answers. Sally Wolper. Wolper Publications, 1983.

The Topic of Cancer. Dick Richards, M.D. England: Pergamon Press, 1982.

Vitamin C Against Cancer. H.L. Newbold, M.D. Stein & Day Publishers, 1979.

Vitamins Against Cancer. Kedar N. Prasad. Nutrition Publishing House, Inc., 1989.

Winning the Fight Against Breast Cancer: The Nutritional Approach. Carlton Fredericks. Grosset & Dunlap, 1979.

World Without Cancer: The Story of Vitamin B17. G. Edward Griffin. American Media, 1980.

QUESTIONNAIRE FOR PATIENTS

It would be extremely helpful if we were able to get some information regarding your experiences with therapies, education programs, support groups, and information organizations. Any information will be confidential if requested, and can be submitted without a name if desired. Such information could be an invaluable service to people like you searching for assistance. Please return the completed questionnaire to the following address: Third Opinion, P.O. Box 50114, Santa Barbara, California 93150.

Name: _____

Address: _____

_____

_____

Patient's name (if different from above): _____

Name of center, program, or service: _____

_____

Location: _____

_____

_____

Attending physician/health care provider: _____

Diagnosis: _____

_____

_____

_____

Treatment: _____

_____

_____

_____

_____

_____

_____

_____

_____

Effectiveness: _____

_____

_____

_____

_____

Length of stay: _____

_____

_____

Cost: _____

_____

Difficulties encountered (if any): _____

_____

_____

_____

_____

_____

Results: _____

_____

_____

_____

_____

_____

Comments: _____

_____

_____

_____

_____

_____

_____

_____

_____

Index